Well To Do

A GUIDE TO TAKE CHARGE, SET GOALS
& IMPROVE YOUR HEALTH

Nicole Eull, Psy.D.

HODI Center Press

Elm Grove, Wisconsin

HODI Center Press
Elm Grove, WI
www.MySkillRx.com

Ordering Information: To purchase print copies please visit amazon.com. For quantity orders of 25 or more, contact us at MySkillRx.com for special pricing.

Well To Do: A Guide to Take Charge, Set Goals & Improve Your Health / Nicole Eull —1st Ed. (rev1)

ISBN **978-1541076402**

Dedicated to my amazing husband. He thought I could, so I did.

Give a skill, not a pill.

—Dr. Nicole Eull

Contents

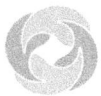

A Note to Primary Care Providers

*This book can help you and your patients set concrete, effective,
and realistic goals that result in real, long-lasting change.*

FOR THE PAST SEVERAL YEARS, I HAVE SERVED AS A FACULTY BEHAVIORIST for a Family Medicine residency program affiliated with the University of Wisconsin. I often have the opportunity to observe young doctors at work as they discuss their patients with a supervising physician. At faculty meetings, my colleagues discuss how they can do more work in less time to try to meet the demands of a competitive marketplace and shrinking reimbursements. I see how frustrated these passionate and caring physicians become when they feel their hard work is just not enough to help patients who are becoming more obese, less active, more chronically ill and more stressed.

My residents look at me with exasperation when I ask them to listen more and spend more time talking to their patients about their behaviors. These new doctors are constantly told to work faster and to fill out more paperwork. Computers freeze up, interpreter phones disconnect without warning, and people show up late for their appointments. In addition to all of this, doctors have stressors of their own. They still have families and pets, school concerts, sick days, leaky faucets, and a second mortgage known as school loans. If they are really doing well, they might also have some hobbies and a social life.

How do you use the twenty, ten or even five minutes that you have with your patients to really make a difference? How do you share with them every journal article, recent study, great book recommendation, and pearl of wisdom you have collected? How do you convince patients to take care of themselves and to accept responsibility for their own health management? How do you set realistic goals, agree on a plan and then hold your patients accountable at their next visit? It's a lot to ask of even the best, most energetic and dedicated physician.

This book is a tool to help you to accomplish this. It emphasizes the patient's position as the head of the project. The patient, after all, has the most to gain from the effort. It provides simple ideas in plain language, in an organized way that most people can understand and relate to. The information is delivered with humor and sometimes my own embarrassing stories. It covers many areas that you encounter regularly with your patients, such as food choices, exercise, sleep, and stress management.

Each chapter ends with a worksheet that provides specific questions and goals for follow up. The book will work best if you first familiarize yourself with the material so that you understand the terms and catch phrases used in the worksheets. These worksheets combine principles of Motivational Interviewing, goal-setting and effective behavioral change techniques to guide you and your patient easily through a productive conversation. Ask your patient to read a chapter that relates to their current health concerns—this will be the patient's homework for the next visit. The patient can also review the worksheet and begin setting personal goals. At your next visit, simply review the worksheet goals together to agree on a realistic plan for the coming weeks or months. Document these goals or save a copy of the worksheet for the next visit. If the goals are met, you can move on to more challenging goals on the same worksheet or move to a new chapter.

The format of this book has several benefits. The first is that it provides a way to organize your thoughts and interventions for a particular health concern. I often find myself remembering a good suggestion after the patient has left. With this book, the ideas are organized in one place. Second, this book can be used as a framework for group visits, which can help you deliver information to patients more efficiently, engaging them in collaboration with you and other patients who understand their struggles. Third, this method of teaching emphasizes the patient's personal responsibility. No matter how committed you are to your work, you probably are not willing to follow your patients home to monitor their nutritional, exercise, and stress management goals. If you finish a medical appointment feeling that you did more work than the patient or you accepted more responsibility than the patient did, then something has gone wrong.

There is much evidence to show that teaching disease self-management skills, such as the ones outlined in these chapters, leads to greater success compared to monitoring and reporting medical markers such as weight and cholesterol. These benefits appear to extend beyond weight loss and improved health markers into quality of life and improved confidence and social engagement. For example, patients are usually keenly aware that they need to lose weight but often don't actually know *how* to lose weight. There is a crucial difference between asking patients whether they are eating healthy and asking them *what they are actually eating*. The first is a yes/no question that is open to a lot of interpretation. The second is a conversation that may reveal serious misconceptions.

My goal with this book is to help you get the conversation started in a way that is organized, time-efficient, and maybe even fun. I welcome any feedback for improvement of future editions of the book and would love to hear how the book is working for you and your patients. You can find additional information and share feedback on my website, **www.MySkillRx.com**.

Primary care practitioners can make a tremendous difference for their patients. I hope this book provides some tools to help your patients make lasting changes that improve and extend their lives.

Live well, work well, teach well,

Nicole

You are In Charge

MY MOTHER HATES WHINERS. She always forbade me to whine as a child. My father always told me, "Don't come to me with problems, come to me with solutions." Thanks to this upbringing I learned to be solution-focused. I learned to look at problems and think about what would make them better. I learned that complaining about things and situations results in zero progress or resolution.

I have to admit, however, that I've spent a lot of time complaining about our current healthcare system. I have spent hours talking with friends and colleagues about this and wondering how anyone survives, much less thrives, in our current state.

Well, I'm finished whining. I'm finished presenting my complaints. This book is my attempt to make a little difference in my corner of healthcare. I have a decade of experience working with primary care doctors. I observe thousands of hours of doctor visits and listen to doctors, physicians' assistants, and nurse practitioners express how frustrated they are trying to genuinely care for people in a rushed clinic and still keep up with mounds of paperwork and other demands.

I also have many family and friends who feel overwhelmed by the massive amounts of information available to them about their health. They struggle to feel connected to anyone who can help them navigate the healthcare system and find the best treatment possible for them. It's so difficult to feel like an individual person with unique needs and priorities.

The good news is that most of the best solutions are really the least expensive and the best defense is a good offense. If you like sports, you can think of this book as your offensive playbook. (My husband will be shocked when he reads this to find I even know what that is.) Otherwise, you can think of this book as the place where you and your doctor set out realistic, clear, and effective strategies to help you feel your best.

My Philosophy

You will notice a few themes in this book:

1. You are in charge.
2. You are not alone.
3. There are no quick fixes.

You Are in Charge

There is very little that your doctors can do to help you if you are not willing to help yourself. They can raise medication dosage and order more tests, but most common health problems these days are caused by lack of movement, too much stress, and unhealthy foods. No doctor can go home with you at night to keep you safe from these things. You have to make a choice to get involved and do your part. Otherwise, doctors are just putting out fires in the clinic while you go home and light more.

You Are Not Alone

The vast majority of doctors and healthcare professionals I know are really good people. They care deeply for their patients and they want to help. My hope is that this book will give you and your doctor a tool that will help you work together in a way that is clear and organized. You may find that just knowing someone is willing to support you is enough to get you motivated. If your doctor is not able to participate in this process, then perhaps you can find a friend or family member to coach you or work through the book at the same time. Think of it as the ultimate book club.

There Are No Quick Fixes

People ask me all the time what supplements, smoothies, and products I recommend for losing weight. My answer is simple: Eat real food in reasonable portions. Move your body. Repeat. Repeat again. And again. Do this most of the time. Enjoy your life. Make friends with people who treat you well. Laugh. There is no product on the market that can give you the same benefits as the above prescription and with the same lasting effects. If one comes out I promise to let you know. The fact is that it takes time and effort to get and stay healthy and anyone who uses the words, "fast," "easy," "quick," or "miracle" is a liar.

How to Use This Book

There are several ways to use this book. One approach is to look through the table of contents and find the chapters that are most important to you. Start with the one that you feel is the most important to your health or talk with your doctor and the two of you can agree on where to begin. Then you can read the chapter and fill out the worksheet or "To Do List" at the end of the chapter. Take this worksheet into your next medical appointment and review your goals with your doctor. Let your provider know what he or she can do to support your goals and keep you accountable for them. You can also review them with a friend or family member to get feedback and encouragement.

Another way to use the book is just as it is written. Start at the beginning and work your way through slowly but surely. Skip the chapters that you don't need. Think of this as a user's manual or a workbook to guide your doctor's visits or your own self-improvement for the next few years.

A Favor

If you like this book and find it useful, please pass it on to someone else. Help me get these solutions out to others. Help me make a big change in small steps, one *To Do List* at a time.

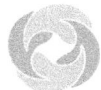

CHAPTER 1

Managing Your Healthcare

A GOOD FRIEND OF MINE HAS STRUGGLED WITH STOMACH PROBLEMS FOR YEARS. There were times when she could barely move because she was in so much pain, and she once spent Christmas on the couch because she was so uncomfortable. Her regular doctors had theories about what could be causing her pain, but no one could say for sure.

For a while she didn't have insurance coverage and years went by with no answers. Eventually she got a job with health insurance and tried to solve the mystery of her terrible stomach pain. She started with one doctor, which led to many doctors, tests and questions. They took lots of blood. They sent her for scans. They asked her multiple times whether she was using cocaine, which she was not. They ran more tests and each set of results led to more tests. She finally became so frustrated that she did not want to look into it any further. She continues to have major stomach problems to the point that sometimes she cannot even eat.

Many of us have health problems that we let go—we ignore them, tolerate them or treat their symptoms without seeking real solutions. There are various reasons why this happens: some of us are afraid of doctors, others are afraid of what the doctor might find, and many of us are put off by the healthcare process of waiting, expensive tests, and more medications. Even when you find a doctor you can trust and might even like, there are so many demands on a doctor's time that you usually only have five to ten minutes to describe your health concerns.

I have spent several years of my career observing medical residents (new doctors in training) in Family Medicine as they work with patients. I observe their appointments, the questions they ask and the recommendations they make, and I provide these new doctors with feedback on their interaction with patients. I have seen some tremendously talented and caring physicians at work, but all of them feel there is not enough time to care for their patients as they wish they could.

This book is for you and your doctor. It provides much of the information you will need to eliminate unhealthy behaviors and begin the work needed to feel healthy, energetic, and focused. I hope you can begin to move beyond confronting your health problems and begin living a healthy and vibrant life. You can think of these chapters as the conversations and ideas that your doctor wishes he or she could share with you, if only there were more time.

The Patient's Job Description

I want to start with a statement that might be a bit controversial. **It is not your doctor's job to make you healthy.** Your doctor can offer you treatments and medicines that may help manage the symptoms of your health problems. A really great doctor can anticipate some conditions you are at risk for and offer ideas and guidelines to help with prevention. But all the real work is in your hands.

Many health concerns that we struggle with today are preventable. Actually, most of them are caused by our unhealthy lifestyle choices. Most of us know this, but we still arrive at medical appointments and look expectantly to our physicians for magical cures to undo the damage we cause ourselves. It's as if we are setting little (and sometimes big) fires all over the house and then looking to the firefighter to put them out so we can set the fires again tomorrow.

In the hospital, I often ask my patients who they think is the boss of their treatment team. They usually guess that it is their doctor or sometimes the nurse for that shift. Others jokingly say, "my wife." They hardly ever name themselves. You are the boss of your healthcare team and that means you are responsible for making sure things are running efficiently in the business of your health and wellness. Your job requirements are listed in our first **Skill Prescription**.

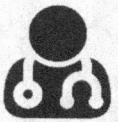 Skill Prescription:

Be the boss of your healthcare

1. Be aware of your health concerns.
2. Know your medications and their side effects.
3. Provide a clear and honest picture of your lifestyle to your healthcare providers.
4. Ask questions in an organized way.
5. Do your own research about your health concerns.
6. Have clear and measurable goals for wellness.
7. Tell your doctor whether the treatment plan you agreed to is working or not.
8. Be prepared to contribute time and effort to meeting your goals.

Be aware of your health concerns

I find it very helpful when patients keep a log or list of their health concerns. This saves a lot of time for both you and your doctor. If the main concerns are clear, you can spend more time developing a plan to target each issue.

It's also helpful to consider how your various health concerns might be related. This is especially important if there are a few things that are causing the majority of the distress. For example, many people are sad, overweight, have diabetes, and high blood pressure. There are many treatments for each of these issues, but there are also some treatments that will help *all* of them. One is exercise and another is eating healthy foods. You can treat every symptom of every disease as its own isolated challenge, or you can look at what's underneath all of those symptoms and start to change your lifestyle.

Know Your Medications and Their Side Effects

If you are prescribed one or two medications for an occasional illness, or you only have a few medications that you take regularly, it's pretty easy to keep track of them. Unfortunately, many patient medication lists have six or more drugs, all with complicated names and an array of side effects and interactions. Whether your list is simple or complicated, it's your responsibility to keep track of what goes into your body and why it's being prescribed. If you can't keep track, then find a friend or family member who can help you.

Keep a list of all of your medications and update it every time a medication is changed (see "My Personal Pharmacy" worksheet at the end of this chapter). Also, pay attention to how you feel in the hours and days after you begin a new medication. Notice whether you feel dizziness, stomach upset, drowsiness, or even irritability, then let your doctor know about these changes. Whenever doctors prescribe a new medication, ask them to explain the reason for it in clear language you understand, and ask them to go through your list with you to ensure the new drug will not interact badly with existing medications you take.

It is also important to keep track of things that have not worked for you in the past, or worse, those medications that have caused problems for you. It seems silly to try a drug that failed in the past, but many people do because they forget what they have already taken. Also, certain people are just more sensitive to medications in general. Have you ever taken a pain pill and felt totally wiped out for the rest of the day? Have you ever reacted with extreme anger or even hallucinations or paranoia when taking a medication? These are things you want to mention to all your doctors so that you can minimize the risk of that happening in the future.

Finally, you'll want to add to this list the vitamins, supplements, and teas that you take at home. Many "herbal remedies" are quite powerful and can interfere with or even amplify other medications. Mention any special creams or other remedies you use on a regular basis. Are you using a humidifier at night? Do you add something to the water? Does your grandma encourage you to take a tea she gets at the Chinese grocery store? Do you use arnica ointment for bruising or buy other natural products when you are sick? Do you take homeopathic tablets? Please let your doctor know.

Provide a Clear and Honest Picture of Your Lifestyle

I'll admit it: I'm prone to embellishing. I've been known to add a little drama to a story for entertainment value, but I don't think I'm alone in this way. Sometimes when I'm at the doctor, I embellish in another way: I provide my doctor the PG-13 version of my health habits. I don't think I *lie* as much as focus on the good things and leave out or downplay a few bad habits. Let's call it *embellishing* my lifestyle description.

The problem is that this doesn't really help anyone. We give our doctors the version of our lives we think they want to hear, or that we wish were true, when the version we need to share is the truth. Our doctors need to know all the ways we promote our health, but they especially need to know the things we need to improve.

I have observed many patients who swear to their doctors that they "eat healthy" and "exercise regularly" when it's not really true. The most difficult situation is when people actually *believe* they are doing the right things but are not.

My advice to both patients and doctors is to **get specific.** When you say, "I eat healthy," what does that mean specifically? How often do you exercise? What kind of exercise do you do? Is that form of exercise something you enjoy? Do you sleep well and how long do you sleep? What time do you go to bed? What do you do to calm down when you are really upset? How much of the day are you feeling happy and comfortable? Do you spend time with nice people who are good to you and make you laugh? Are you having any fun? Do you spend most nights in front of the TV or are you doing meaningful and healthy activities? Do you sit down for meals? Do you share meals with your family? Do you engage in some activity you consider spiritual or healing? Are you smoking, drinking, or doing drugs? How much caffeine do you drink?

It is so important that you tell your doctor all the good stuff <u>and</u> the bad stuff. Yes, you might get a lecture. But the fact is, you might need a lecture. For some of us, the more times we hear that things could be better, the more likely we are to consider making a change. Maybe hearing yourself saying it out loud will be upsetting enough to help you make an attitude shift.

Ask Questions in an Organized Way

I used to leave the doctor's office and immediately realize that I forgot to ask some important question. I usually remembered even more questions as the day continued. Now, when I have a doctor's appointment coming up for myself or my children, I start a list of questions in my cell phone or write them down in a place that's easy to get to. This way I have them ready the day of the appointment and I feel more satisfied with my experience. This is even more important when you have many health concerns.

I used to work in a pain clinic in the county hospital in Chicago. Most of my patients were in constant pain, in addition to dealing with other stressors like poverty and mental illness. I started teaching my patients this simple idea of being prepared for their doctor's appointments, and I noticed a few things. Patients felt more organized and in control of their healthcare and their appointments. They also felt less confused and more informed.

What I didn't expect was how much the doctors appreciated it and how their perceptions of the patients changed. They started to describe the list-making patients as organized, hardworking, and taking responsibility for their health. I believe they enjoyed working with these patients more and were excited about giving them the best treatment possible. The doctors also felt these patients valued the limited time they were able to spend. It's likely that patients who take an *active* and *organized* role in their healthcare will enjoy much better outcomes, for all of these reasons.

Do Your Own Research

"Ignorance is bliss," we say, but that kind of bliss only lasts for a little while. It's so important that you understand your health concerns. Some people are naturally curious and will go online the second they receive a new diagnosis. Some may feel overwhelmed by the amount of information available. One major problem is that much of the health information you find online, in magazines or on TV is exaggerated or just plain false.

Where do you go for good information? I would suggest you start with your doctor. Specialists read lots of books and other materials on the diseases in which specialize. They may know of a good book written by someone with a particular disease or one written by a specialist in layperson's terms.

The next place I would recommend is your nearest hospital library. In the hospital system where I work, every hospital has a library staffed by amazingly talented and intelligent medical librarians. These professionals can put together a list of easily understood resources for you to read, and they can help you check them out for free. If you don't have the time or desire to read, some libraries also carry videos and CDs about many different topics.

The internet is both a wonderful and a terrible resource. I suggest that you start with the sites below for reliable information that is user-friendly and easy to read:

- Mayo Clinic: www.mayoclinic.com/health-information
- Cleveland Clinic: my.clevelandclinic.org/health

- WebMD: www.webmd.com
- National Center for Complementary and Alternative Medicine: www.nccam.nih.gov

National associations for particular diseases can be great resources, too. Just search online for your health concern and scan the results for an organization dedicated to serving people with the problem. Well-known and reputable examples include the American Diabetes Association (www.diabetes.org) and the American Cancer Society (www.cancer.org). But it's not only these common diseases—you'll be amazed what rare conditions have a national association. These sites can also help you find doctors, products and research related to the disease. One caution: You may want to read blogs or chat rooms related to a disease with a skeptical eye. Remember that blog posts and comments often reflect only the experiences of one person—a person who is different from you.

Not everyone has access to the internet. Remember that almost all libraries have computers you can use for free, ways to print for a low cost, and librarians who can help you learn to search for information. Most hospitals and hospital libraries also have free internet access. Don't be afraid to ask for help.

Doing your own research can lead to some frightening results. Especially on the internet, you're likely to come across scary stories that may or may not be true, and could be very rare or uncommon. If you're afraid, tell your doctor about your fears. Ask your doctor about the latest research that might affect you and ask him or her to explain these things in words that you understand. Your doctors can serve you much better if they know your concerns.

Have Clear and Measurable Goals

When you want to improve your health, start with the problem that concerns you the most. Figure out one behavior that you can add or take away to address this problem, and put it into a **measurable** goal. Then you and your doctor will have some way to know that you have met your goal.

When I was working on my thesis in graduate school, I would write "work on thesis" in my calendar almost every Saturday and Sunday morning. I'd wake up on the weekends, look at that phrase, feel totally overwhelmed, and then have a minor panic attack and go back to bed. Needless to say, my thesis was not coming along very well.

The solution to my problem was almost comical. My university asked me to teach a class in how to complete a thesis. How ironic! I started researching how to organize information and I came across a great analogy: Compare your task to a marathon. (Now, I'm never going to run a marathon, but I found the comparison very helpful.) If I wanted to run a marathon, I would definitely not start off running the full length of a marathon—26.2 miles. Let's say I plan to run the marathon one year from now. To reach that goal, I would plan so in six months I'm able to run about 13 miles. In three months, I would need to be able to run 6.5 miles. Within the first month, I only need to be able to run two miles, and tomorrow I only need to try on my running shoes. Trying on shoes sounds a lot easier than running 26 miles, doesn't it?

I applied this theory to my thesis and started to progress much faster. I started to write smaller tasks in the calendar like, "Find 10 useful articles" or, "read two articles and take notes." These tasks seemed so much more reasonable and my anxiety disappeared almost completely. The other benefit is that I knew when I was done with the task for the day because I could measure or count it.

You can also do this with health goals. Perhaps your doctor thinks you should be walking 30 minutes a day, and maybe you think that sounds nearly impossible. Could you start with 10 minutes three times a week? Every week you could add five minutes or one more day. This way you are always making progress but you don't feel totally overwhelmed.

Provide Feedback to Your Doctor

I'm pretty sure my doctor is not psychic. She's amazing, but not quite that amazing. I also don't think she has me come to see her so we can have a polite conversation in which I protect her feelings. My doctor wants me to be honest with her about what is working and what is not working.

It's very important that you tell your doctor what is working for you. There are so many paths to healing, and a treatment that works well for one person may result in bad side effects for another person. You are an individual and your treatment needs to be individualized to you.

Be Prepared to Contribute Time and Effort to Your Goals

Your health will not improve without some effort from you. If you believe in miracles and the power of prayer, then pray for the strength and resolve you need to make a positive change. You know the saying, "God helps those who help themselves?" Most religions acknowledge that you are a major part of your own healing. Your health also will not improve just because you go to the doctor frequently. Nearly all health concerns improve through your own effort. That can include getting to treatments, taking your medications consistently, moving your body, or eating well. It may mean all of these things. Remember, you are the boss of your healthcare team, and it is your job to improve your health.

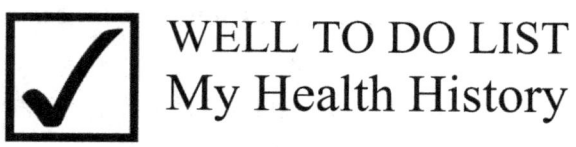 WELL TO DO LIST
My Health History

Medical History

Immediate Health Concerns:

_____

_____

Chronic Health Conditions:

_____

_____

Previous Illnesses:
Major, recurring or uncommon illnesses, including those in childhood

_____

_____

Surgeries:

_____

_____

Response to Surgery:

_____

_____

My Personal Pharmacy

Current Prescription Medications:

Medication	Dose	Recommended Frequency	Reason for Use	Actual Use *How often do you actually take it?*

Current Over-the-Counter Medications:

Include pain relievers like aspirin or ibuprofen, herbs, supplements, vitamins, teas, tinctures, creams, ointments, and other treatment products you use regularly.

Medication	Dose	Recommended Frequency	Reason for Use	Actual Use *How often do you actually take it?*

Past Medications:

Medication	Dose	Frequency of Use	Reason for Use	Reason & Date Stopped

What do you take or do when you have a headache?

_____

What do you take or do when you have a cold?

_____

What do you take or do when your stomach is upset?

_____

What do you take or do when you are in pain?

_____

What do you take or do when you are tired?

_____

What do you take or do when you are angry?

_____

What do you take or do when you are sad?

_____

What do you take or do when you can't sleep?

Health Goals

Things I would like to change/improve in the next month:

_____

_____

_____

Things I would like to change/improve in the next year:

_____

_____

_____

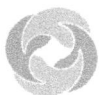

CHAPTER 2

Get Healthy, Stay Healthy: Changing Behaviors

IF IT WERE EASY TO CHANGE BEHAVIORS, there wouldn't be a whole section of self-help books in every bookstore across the country. However, I think it's actually harder to *decide* to change a behavior than it is to actually change it. If you're like most people, you waste tons of time and energy avoiding change. This energy could just as easily be directed to making yourself better. **The first step is to decide that you are really ready to change.** Save yourself and your doctor a lot of frustration by being honest about this.

I had a patient a few years ago who came to me for help with an eating disorder. We tried everything. We worked on changing habits. We used hypnosis and meditation. She started new hobbies to avoid binging and she worked with other practitioners as well. One day she came to her session and said she wasn't planning on coming back. I didn't blame her since I hadn't really been of any help. She bravely admitted that she just wasn't ready to change. She felt that her eating issues hadn't become enough of a problem to move her to stop. I felt that I had failed her, but I appreciated her honesty with me, and most importantly with herself.

Stages of Change

The Stages of Change Model was developed many years ago by psychology researchers James Prochaska and Carlo DiClemente. This useful approach can help you figure out how ready you are to make the changes you need to be a healthier and happier person. The Stages of Change Model divides readiness to change into six stages.

- The first, *Pre-contemplation,* is the stage in which you are not ready to change at all. In fact, you probably don't even see your behaviors as a problem.
- The next stage is *Contemplation.* Now you are recognizing that things are not working well and you are starting to think about making some improvements in your life.
- The third stage is *Preparation.* In this stage you begin to make plans and develop strategies to add new healthy behaviors and/or get rid of unhealthy behaviors.
- The fourth stage is *Action.* Now you are really moving along and have started enacting your plan for change.
- The fifth stage is *Maintenance.* At this point, your new way of living has become more of a habit and doesn't seem like so much work. It might take two weeks or two years to get to this point.
- The sixth stage, unfortunately, is *Relapse.* Let's hope you don't have to deal with this stage, but it happens. It's best to have a relapse prevention plan as soon as you start making improvements. That way stressful situations won't sneak up on you and drive you back to old habits.

You and your doctor should be focusing on different things depending on where you are in the stages of change. The **Skill Prescription** chart below can help you target your efforts and move yourself through the stages of change more quickly.

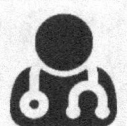

Skill Prescription:

Identify Your Stage of Change & Focus

Stage of Change	Focus
Pre-contemplation *"Problem? What problem?"*	• Continue to evaluate the need for change and listen to your doctor with an open mind. • Understand the risks and how they personally affect you.
Contemplation *"Houston, we have a problem."*	• Explore the pros and cons of change. • Surround yourself with people who make you believe you should and can change.
Preparation *"What's the plan?"*	• Talk to your doctor or friends about how to change safely. • Be honest about things that might get in the way and make plans to avoid these things. • Begin gathering friends who want to help. • Make realistic goals.
Action *"Today is the day!"*	• Start with easy steps. • Replace bad stress management behaviors with good ones. • Believe in yourself or spend time with people who do. • Reward yourself for progress.
Maintenance *"Keep up the good work!"*	• Have a plan for preventing relapse. • Continue to reward yourself. • Explore new things you can do with your new healthier body and mind.
Relapse *"That chocolate bar attacked me when I wasn't looking," or "I give up."*	• Forgive yourself and get back on track. • Learn from your mistakes. • Improve stress management and self-care.

A Change in Perspective

Recently I came home from work after a very long and tiring day. The entire month had been full of non-stop activity and I was cranky and exhausted. Unfortunately, I also had to teach yoga that night. I imagine most people prefer their yoga teacher to appear calm and energetic instead of anxious and tired, so I was not in the best frame of mind to teach.

What I really wanted was to sit on the couch, watch TV and drink a glass of wine - maybe throw in some junk food too, just to top it off. I was walking through my house thinking these thoughts to myself when I realized how terrible it sounded: *"I feel tired and anxious so I want to sit around and eat junk that will make me feel more tired and anxious."* Not the best plan I've ever come up with, and certainly not what I teach my patients and students.

Instead, I took some time to try to adjust my attitude. What I came up with is "I feel tired and anxious and what I need is to teach this yoga class because the movement will make me feel calmer, and my students always make me feel energetic and appreciated." After convincing myself of that message, I went to teach. By the end of the class, I felt great.

One of my college professors introduced me to the concept below. It's a simple graph in which one line (up and down) is a continuum from calm to anxious, and the crossing line (left to right) is a continuum from tired to energetic.

Anxious Tired	Anxious Energetic
Calm Tired	Calm Energetic

- ANXIETY +

- ENERGY +

Unfortunately, I think many of us spend a lot of time in the Anxious/Tired box. That's not a place anyone really wants to be. Sometimes it's good to be Calm/Tired. It's ideal to be in this box when you are ready to sleep. I might need to be a little Anxious/Energetic when I have a deadline or I have to speak in front of a group. It's always best if I feel Calm/Energetic when I sit down to write.

What I love about this diagram is that it helps me think about my goals. If I'm feeling Calm/Tired but I have to write treatment notes, how do I move to Calm/Energetic? Most of us tend to grab a cup of coffee. That may give us some energy, but it may also make us feel anxious. A better way to move to that box might be to get up and walk around a bit before sitting down to the computer.

What if you have worked all day and are feeling Anxious/Tired? That's not the best way to start your evening. You might yell at the kids or have a poor night of sleep. How do you get to Calm/Tired? A slow walk might help, or listening to relaxing music. Maybe you have a good book to read, or you might enjoy talking to a friend who is reassuring and makes you laugh.

The main idea here is to pause to feel where you are right now. Then decide where you want or need to be right now. Finally you need to be honest, and maybe a little creative, to figure out how you can get to where you need to be in a healthy way.

Making Change That Lasts

My guess is that if you are reading this chapter, then you have already decided that something needs to change. Maybe you want to lose weight or want to stop smoking. Perhaps you want to yell less at your kids or wear lipstick more often. The specific behavior you want to change, eliminate or improve is up to you, but this chapter can help you get there while still having some fun.

Step 1: Be Clear About What You Want

What is it that you really hope to accomplish? Do you want to lose weight or do you want to feel more energy? Maybe you want to fit into your clothes again, or you are hoping to prevent diabetes or heart disease. It really helps you and your doctor if you can make your goals relevant and important to you. Some people *say* they want to lose weight because they *think* that is what their doctor wants to hear. The same person might be really motivated by the thought of walking pain-free or feeling more relaxed and sleeping better. Knowing what motivates you helps others encourage you and help you meet your goals. It also helps you identify rewards for good behavior that are tempting and appropriate (see Step 6).

Step 2: Set Specific and Measurable Goals

"I want to be healthier!"

That sounds like a great idea, but what the heck does it mean? I want you to break that down for me: How will I know when you have become "healthier?" You and your doctor should be able to <u>measure</u> your progress and to know when you have actually accomplished something. Many patients come to appointments and tell me that they feel "better." That sounds pretty good, but I want to know specifically *in what way* they are better.

I had an amazing patient recently. When she came in for her first session, we identified a lot of good things she was doing, but she was not doing any exercise. This was especially concerning since she also mentioned that she was often feeling angry, resentful, and impatient. I explained to her that exercise is a great way to burn off anxiety and stress and often helps people manage anger. At the following session, I was thrilled to hear that she had started attending her gym regularly. Even more exciting was the fact that she was able to describe three different times when she noticed a difference in her attitude at work. She was certain this was directly due to her new exercise regimen.

"Back It Up and Break It Down"

I often teach new doctors this phrase: "Back it up and break it down." What I mean is that doctors and patients should make goals one at a time, define progressions, and make sure they can measure progress. First, divide the goal into something that doesn't feel so overwhelming (see the marathon example in Chapter 1 for more details). Specify a *what* and a *how* for the goal. "I want to lose weight" is a *what*. "I want to exercise more" is a *how*. "I want to prevent health problems" is a *what*. "I want to stop smoking" is a *how*.

Each *what* needs to have a *how,* and we need to make that *how* specific. If you want to cut down on how much soda you drink, you might reduce your soda intake by one can/bottle per week. If you want to improve your relationship with your spouse or partner, you might start by making time every week for a date night, or start by talking to each other rather than reading the paper at breakfast. These are things that you can count and check. They are also things that don't feel so big and scary.

"I'm Not Buying What You're Selling"

I don't think people mean to lie to me, but I don't ever believe them when they use absolute statements like "I'm going to cut out *all* carbs," or "I'm *never* going to say mean things about my sister again." Oh, please! Carbs are tasty. Sometimes your sister deserves some criticism. The idea is to live a better and healthier life, not to be perfect. We're just real people trying to do our best.

Let's be more realistic. Before you change that problematic behavior, you should already be thinking of the things that will get in the way. I used to say that I was going to write this book in the hours after my daughter went to bed. That's an admirable goal. The reality is that I always fall asleep if I sit still for longer than 10 minutes after 8 p.m. I finally had to accept that all my most useful thoughts occur before noon and it pretty much goes downhill from there. So my goal became to write for two to three hours one to two times per week. I even started to set dates and mark off space in my calendar for writing.

Take your general goals. Turn them into behaviors. Break that down further into what you can do today. Make sure that you can measure what you have done. Make sure you can measure your progress over time. Finally, make sure this is something you can integrate into your life forever and not just for a little while.

Step 3: Have Some Fun

I hate treadmills. I think they're boring and they make me feel like a hamster. Another thing I hate with a passion is running. I love watching people run and I imagine myself in cute running gear, zooming down the road while the fat flies off my body. What I actually look like running is much more disturbing and I hope you never have to see it. What I love to do is yoga and anything that involves other people and good music. My exercise schedule has to include the things I love. I am always more motivated to be around other people than to work out in my basement.

I had a patient who refused to work out. He had a million reasons why he had no time or place to exercise. I kept encouraging him, but he wouldn't budge. One day I found out that he was a passionate bowler. The man lit up when he talked about bowling. I asked him if he would be willing to walk the length of the bowling alley in between each of his turns on league nights. He agreed. This helped him to start moving and it also reduced the amount of beer and snacks he consumed. It was a start.

Another patient would binge eat when she was bored. I found out that she had always thought about being a writer, and I encouraged her to sign up for a writing class. She noticed right away when she was working on her assignments for the class, she had much less anxiety and wasn't thinking about food as much.

One of my patients was spending many hours caring for a family member who was very ill. He needed to get out of the house. He was a very intelligent man and he needed to be challenged mentally. In one session, he mentioned that he would like to improve his Spanish. I connected him with a Spanish practice group in the area and he joined right away. The group helped him improve his social life and exercise his brain as well.

I think it's important to use our passions to help motivate behaviors. For my professional license I have to attend 20 hours of continuing education every year, but I make sure that the topics are ones that really excite me. Outside of work, I'm really passionate about food and I love to cook. In an effort to eat healthier, I treat myself to healthy cooking classes a couple of times a year.

Step 4: Use Peer Pressure

How many of you look back at your high school pictures and wonder how you could have possibly thought you were cool? How many of you have done really stupid things to impress your friends? How many of you still do this? I have so many patients who started smoking because their friends were doing it. Others drink too much because that's the only way they know how to interact with their friends.

Peer pressure can work in a positive way as well. Other people can encourage you to meet your goals. People can help each other. It is much easier to get up in the morning and take that walk if you know Betty is down the street waiting for you. Truth be told, Betty is only getting up because she knows you will be on your way.

Surround yourself with people who make you feel happy and make you want to be a better and healthier person. You can probably think of a few right now. Tell these people what your goals are so they can help keep you on task toward meeting these goals.

What about the people who don't want you to change? What if that person is your spouse or parent? Many of my patients with diabetes tell me that they have to keep explaining to their families why they cannot have birthday cake or share a jumbo box of candy at the movies. Be patient. These people are not as far along on the stages of change. Lead by example. Often, when these people see how happy you are and how much fun you are having, they may want to know more about your success. You may start to provide positive peer pressure for them. Think of yourself as a trendsetter and enjoy watching your success multiply.

Step 5: Post Reminders

Another way to keep focused on your task or goal is to set up reminders throughout the places that you live and work. A friend of mine played college basketball, and her team's sports psychologist encouraged the players to write their goals on sticky notes and place them all around their homes. My friend feels this helped her change the way she saw herself. As she read the messages every day, they started to sink in and become part of her. During the two years she did this practice, she was an All-Big Ten shooting guard. (I don't know exactly what that means, but my husband tells me it's impressive.)

Step 6: Reward Yourself

Maybe you want more energy so you can keep up with your kids. When you start exercising more, you might reward yourself with a fun outing with your children. Perhaps you want to quit smoking so your things won't smell anymore. In that case, you might want to get your carpet cleaned or buy a few new outfits for yourself after you are smoke-free for two months. My mother once offered to pay for a manicure if my cousin could stop biting her nails for one month. It worked.

We seem to know instinctively that children need rewards to motivate them to do things, but somehow don't think that we as adults need rewards. Of course we do! We work because our jobs are meaningful and interesting at best, or at least provide a paycheck. We spend time with people who make us feel good or make us laugh. We often work harder for people who express appreciation or pride in the work we do. Our children drive us crazy, but we keep loving them because of those occasions when they snuggle in and give us a hug that melts everything else away.

We are wired to respond to rewards. We can use this knowledge to shape our own behaviors and the behaviors of others. I used to complain constantly about Monday Night Football. My husband has learned a thing or two by living with a psychologist, so he started giving me neck massages during the game. Soon I began to look forward to football. Well, "look forward to football" might be a stretch, but at least I didn't complain anymore.

Part of a good plan for long-term change is making sure that you have a great system of rewards in place to keep you motivated. It also makes things much more fun.

Step 7: Forgive and Move Forward

Keep in mind that these behaviors you want to change might not go quietly. They may fight to stick around and reappear when you least expect them. Habits are hard to change. When old habits reappear, you might feel like a failure or start to criticize yourself harshly. Don't be too hard on yourself or you may destroy the confidence needed to continue with growth and change. It's best to expect some slip-ups at times, but you want to avoid using the slip-up as an excuse to give up completely. Don't "forgive and forget." In this case, it's better to "forgive, learn, and keep going."

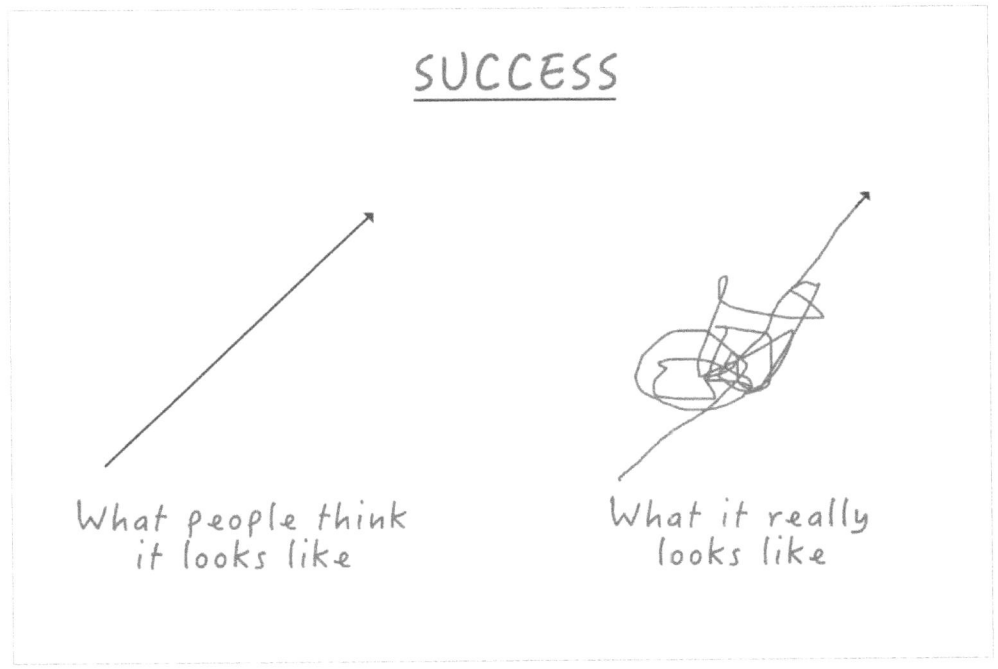

Concept credited to actor/comedian Demetri Martin's book, This Is a Book (Grand Central, 2011).

Let Your Doctor Know

There are many small and easy changes that you can start making today. I just want to remind you to invite your doctor to be part of any changes that involve your physical and mental health. He or she may have some great ideas or resources that can get you started. Your doctor will also be able to tell you if there are any health concerns with your plan.

For example, there are many people who come to me hoping to reduce or eliminate their medications. I think that's a great goal, but there are many medications that have to be reduced slowly or you may become sick. Along those lines, it's always good to exercise more, but an increase in exercise might require some changes in medications for diabetes, for example. There is a lot of evidence that exercise can actually reduce chronic pain, but there may be certain kinds of exercise that would be safer than others. Involving your doctor will only increase the amount of support and encouragement you'll have to make these changes permanent.

✔ WELL TO DO LIST
Making Changes that Last

What is the behavior I want to focus on changing?

_____

Why do I want to change?

_____

What stage of change am I in? (Circle one)

    Pre-contemplation   Preparation   Maintenance

    Contemplation   Action   Relapse

Set a SMART Goal:

  Specific: What exactly am I going to change?

  _____

  Measurable: How will I know that the goal is accomplished?

  _____

  Actionable: What are the behaviors I am going to do?

  _____

  Realistic: Is this something I can accomplish by the date I have set?

  _____

  Time-limited: When will I accomplish this goal?

  _____

How can I make this fun?

_____

_____

Who will help me meet this goal?

How will I remind myself of my goal?

How will I reward myself when my goal is met?

Will my doctor need to make any changes to my medications or treatments based on this change?

CHAPTER 3

Eating in a Modern World

I THINK THE BIGGEST PROBLEM WITH WEIGHT LOSS is the idea of going on "diets." Our society focuses so much on fad diets and quick fixes. There are millions of teas, pills, supplements, and foods that are supposed to make weight loss easy. These are lies. There is no quick and effortless way to get and stay healthy. It takes effort and discipline. This may sound discouraging, but it also means that you don't have to go to extremes to be healthy and fit. You just have to make a few good choices every day.

Cravings

We all start out with the best of intentions. We tell ourselves that we will eat healthy and then those cravings set in. Suddenly, your mind is consumed with thoughts of sweets and salty junk food and you can barely concentrate on anything else.

When you give in to your cravings, do you feel bad about yourself afterwards? I do. I pride myself on being a disciplined person with a fair amount of willpower. I have cut out doughnuts, soda, artificial sweeteners . . . lots of the fun stuff. However, I sometimes find myself at the drive-in ordering a chocolate shake or at parties leaning over the chip bowl with crumbs flying everywhere, growling at anyone who threatens to take some for themselves. If only I were exaggerating. You should see me with a bowl of movie popcorn. It's troubling.

I've been learning a lot about cravings lately. It's actually pretty interesting, because it seems we have biology to blame. When you get stressed out once in a while, your body recovers pretty quickly if you take care of yourself. Unfortunately, most of us function in a constant state of stress. Our bodies don't have time to recover and the chemistry of our bodies actually changes. The chemicals that are meant to help us through emergencies increase and the chemicals that keep us calm and relaxed start to decrease.

One important chemical is called serotonin. Serotonin is the "feel good" chemical in our body and brain. It's like the Bob Marley inside us singing, "Don't worry about a thing." Interestingly, it's also one of the chemicals that keep us feeling calm and rational enough to avoid unhealthy foods. Serotonin is in lots of places in the body. One place it hangs out is around the *prefrontal cortex*, which is the part of our brain that gives us impulse control. It's the part of your brain that keeps you from telling your boss that he or she is an idiot even if it would feel good to say it. When serotonin gets low, the prefrontal cortex does not run as well, and you may find yourself in an unemployment line wishing you had kept your mouth shut.

Scientists are now discovering that serotonin also hangs out near our stomachs. When serotonin is low, your stomach can react to stress by signaling the brain that there is an emergency and that you are going to need lots of fuel (in the form of Doritos and pizza) to run away from danger. So now you have your stomach begging for quick sugars and your self-control is out the window.

Another thing that can reduce the levels of serotonin in your body is the sugary and fattening foods themselves. That's a double whammy. The unhealthy food makes you more likely to crave unhealthy food in the future. There are certain companies that actually engineer foods in a lab to do this. (Some of these companies can be recognized by the drive-thru lane and dollar menu at their restaurants.) It's depressing to see how much worse this gets over time if you continue to consume these foods. It's much better to avoid these foods in the first place.

The good news is that there are many foods that actually increase levels of serotonin in your brain and body. See Chapter 4 for more details on these real, fresh, colorful, and varied foods that are in their natural form, or close to it. These foods are naturally high in vitamins and minerals and they make you feel great. If you eat a meal and feel tired and mentally slow afterwards, that reaction tells you that those foods aren't good for you. When you eat a meal and feel energized and happy, you know you have found your perfect fuel.

Portion Control

There are a lot of suggestions out there for how to limit your portions. Some nutritionists and doctors can give you helpful suggestions about exactly how much of each food group you should be eating at each meal and snack. I'm not a nutritionist, but I will offer you a few ideas to get you started.

First, at mealtime, try using a smaller salad plate instead of a full-sized dinner plate. This way you just don't have the space to pile on that pasta you love so much. Also, keep in mind that restaurants are terrible places for portion control. They normally serve way too much for one meal. I suggest asking for a to-go container right away with your meal and putting half of your serving away for later before you even start eating. Out of sight, out of mind. The added benefit here is that lunch is already made for tomorrow.

Another suggestion is to make sure your plate is colorful. This usually requires fruits and vegetables and a mix of different foods, ensuring that your body gets a variety of nutritional resources to draw on. Another option is to make a rule in the house that you have to wait 15 minutes before going back for seconds. This will give the family more time to talk and catch up on the day, and by then your stomach will have time to let your brain know it is full.

Mindful Eating

How many times have you finished a meal and realized you don't remember eating it? Have you ever started a bag of chips in front of the television and then realized you had eaten the whole bag? What about feeling the need to "clean your plate" without paying attention to whether you are actually still hungry? In our rushed society, we are always trying to multi-task and meals rarely get their own dedicated time. This means that we are often eating while driving to work, paying bills, talking on the phone or surfing the internet.

Being mindful means being totally engaged in the present moment. You are much more likely to enjoy your food, eat the right amount, and choose the right kinds of food if you are paying attention. This means there should be a time set aside for eating, at a table, with a plate, and with no electronic devices within reach. This includes the television. Take the time to really taste your food. If you taste each bite then you are likely to feel more satisfied and eat less. There is some evidence to show that your body may even better digest the food you eat if you are paying attention to the experience.

Family Dinners

Growing up my family always ate dinner together. We even took turns cooking. By age eleven, I had my own night to plan the evening meal. That's not to say that everything we ate together was particularly healthy, and it usually wasn't made from scratch or organic, but we were nurtured by each other's company and we knew the details of each other's lives.

There are many reasons to encourage families to eat dinner together. Numerous studies point to the benefits for children. Children who live in homes where the family eats dinner together the majority of the time are less likely to smoke, drink, do drugs, get depressed, develop eating disorders and consider suicide. They are also more likely to do well in school, delay having sex, eat healthier foods and learn social graces. It also seems that families who eat together regularly have less tension and more intimate conversation.

There are benefits for adults, too. This is a wonderful way to reconnect with your family and to know what challenges and joys your loved ones are experiencing. It's also a time to set aside stress and resentment from the day and to eat in a mindful way. You are more likely to enjoy your meal, feel satisfied, and avoid later snacking.

This practice is good for any kind of family, not just traditional families. Even if you don't have children at home, and even if you live alone, there is still value in making a ritual out of mealtime. Turn off the TV, take your time, and think of your meal as an opportunity for spiritual nourishment rather than just another chore.

Every evening meal can be a small celebration of the many blessings that we experience throughout the day. Every dinner provides time for you to nurture your family and yourself.

Live It Up

Have you ever noticed that well-made food seems to fill you up better than junk? I can eat a whole bag of tortilla chips and still be hungry, but a nourishing meal can be served in small portions and I feel satisfied. Our bodies recognize real food and use it much more effectively than processed junk foods. It's true. There are lots of books and articles written about Mediterranean diets, or why French women don't get fat, and you can read them for more details. You are not reading this book for overly detailed information about soluble fats and triglycerides. You just want to look good and feel healthy.

I think the true beauty of some of the more popular holistic eating plans recommended by health professionals is that they emphasize filling, healthy, diverse and even pretty food that tastes delicious in a natural state. These diets also emphasize quality of life by eating slowly and trying new foods while consuming things that give energy rather than taking it away.

What's the Plan, Stan?

Most of us feel that life keeps getting busier and crazier. This leaves a lot of us in a position where we don't have time to cook healthy meals for ourselves or our families. This is where you have to plan ahead. There are a couple of things you can do to make sure that you are not stuck with limited, unhealthy options.

Let's start with the grocery store. Don't you dare go there hungry, or you will come home with twice as much as you need and most of it will be junk. Plan your meals for the week ahead of time, and when you do go to the store, take a list that reflects the meals you have planned. Meal planning and good decisions at the store set the foundation for your eating the rest of the week.

The main enemy of healthy eating is junk food. The key to controlling the supply of junk food is not bringing it home in the first place. I can usually avoid chips because I don't buy them, but if they are left after a party you can bet my husband and I will eat the whole bag, including the crumbs.

It's worse if there is chocolate in the house. I'll think about it constantly until it's gone. Rather than buy junk food and then try to limit your consumption, make the decision at the store not to bring it home. When you have to work harder to get it, you're less likely to eat it.

What about snacks? It's recommended to eat three healthy meals and two to three small, healthy snacks throughout the day. This is a much better way to lose weight than skipping meals because, when you don't eat, your metabolism gets slower and slower, meaning you burn fewer calories. When you have healthy snacks with you, your body can stay energized and your brain can stay alert. Things like fruit, fresh veggies, nuts, seeds, nut butters, cheese, whole-grain crackers, or plain popcorn can all fuel the body. Cookies, chips, and other processed foods will add fat and sugar to your diet and make you feel tired. Juice will give you a temporary sugar rush without the good fiber of fruit. Those convenient granola bars are often very high in sugar and artificial ingredients. Take the time to read the ingredients and nutritional information on your foods. Prepare healthy snacks at the start of the day and make sure you eat a little bit every few hours. Have the good stuff with you and you will be less tempted to eat the junk.

Getting Started

As with any self-improvement, changing your diet can be a challenge. We all start out with the best intentions but seem to go back to the usual routine within a few weeks or even a few hours. My patients often want to take on everything that I suggest at the same time. It's so common that I have started limiting what I tell people in the first session. It's best to make *small* changes, and make them *one at a time*. If you would like some ideas of how to approach change in an organized and realistic way, see Chapter 2 on making changes.

More Bang for Your Buck

The bottom line is this: Eat real foods. Can you identify how it was made or where it came from? Would a person from 200 years ago recognize it as food? Do you truly feel full and satisfied after a reasonable portion? If you can follow even some of the suggestions above, you will probably be thinner, nicer, calmer, happier, healthier, and more energetic. That's a pretty sweet deal!

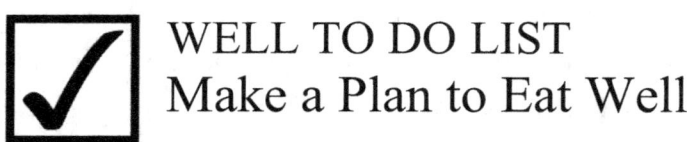

WELL TO DO LIST
Make a Plan to Eat Well

Circle five of these foods that you can start eating this month:

Happy Foods ☺ - eat these foods to boost your mood and curb cravings.

brown rice

whole-grain cereals

salmon

fresh tuna

sardines

chicken *(grilled or baked)*

turkey

walnuts

flax seeds

sunflower seeds

pumpkin seeds

sesame seeds

almonds

cashews

egg whites

milk

yogurt

bananas

kiwi

pineapple

plantains

plums

grapefruit

mango

honeydew melon

cantaloupe

tomatoes

avocado

corn

broccoli

cauliflower

green leafy vegetables
(spinach, greens, kale, collards, etc.)

baked potatoes with skin

mushrooms

cooked beans
(kidney, pinto, lentils, chickpeas, etc.)

Which skill will you work on this month?

Use a smaller plate

Eat mindfully

Limit seconds

Make a more colorful plate

Sit down with the family for meals

Set aside distractions

List one food you will not eat this month:
Examples: soda, candy, doughnuts, chips, fried food

_____

List one food you will eat less of this month:

List a healthy snack you can eat…

at home: _____

at work: _____

on the go: _____

Consider foods that are have just a few basic ingredients and are minimally packaged and processed such as a handful of nuts, a piece of fruit, plain yogurt, hummus and carrots, or a hard boiled egg.

CHAPTER 4

The Best Food for You

When diet is wrong, medicine is of no use. When diet is correct, medicine is of no need.

—ancient Ayurvedic proverb

MOST OF US START TO REALLY LOOK AT OUR FOOD CHOICES when we get concerned about our weight. The first things we think of to control our weight are diet and exercise. I will touch on exercise in a later chapter because it's clearly important, but weight issues start with what you eat. Exercise will not undo the damage of unhealthy, fattening and toxic food, and eating these bad foods will often make it impossible to have the energy to exercise. The importance of food goes way beyond weight, impacting mental and physical health more than anything else we do. Let's start by talking about how to feed your body and mind with premium fuel for maximum performance.

Quality Control

As the hospitalized patients I work with begin to prepare to go home, I review four things that will help prevent anxiety and depression. I tell them to eat well, sleep well, move (exercise), and have fun every day. I always start with food because it is so important to how our bodies function. I usually give people a few options to guide their food choices. You can decide which ones you can manage.

When considering food choices and purchasing habits, some people say they can't afford the healthier options, whether in dollars or time. When evaluating real food versus quicker, unhealthy options, I encourage you to consider the cost of health problems, lack of energy, and time spent dealing with the consequences of unhealthy eating. When you consider the whole picture, healthy food choices look much more affordable.

Real Food

The first recommendation is to buy most of your food from the outside ring of the grocery store, because that's where you find the real food. How many ingredients are in a tomato? Exactly one, last time I counted. Things like dairy products, meats, vegetables, fruits, and seafood are simple foods and are less likely to be as processed as the "food" that is canned, boxed, shrink-wrapped, and dried in the center aisles.

Don't get me wrong. I have a busy life and a picky toddler, so I buy frozen foods smashed into the shape of dinosaurs, and God bless macaroni and "cheese" when I just don't have anything left to give. But I make an effort to have these be the exception, not the usual—the 20 percent, not the 80. The idea is to eat food most of the time that is as close to its natural form and as simple as possible.

Here's another idea. Some people try to limit their purchases to things that have five ingredients or less. Others try to limit purchases to only things with ingredients they can pronounce. If it sounds like it came from a lab, it probably did, and if you don't recognize an ingredient, your body probably won't either. Our bodies are meant to use things found in nature and not labs.

Local Food

I can go on forever about my passion for local foods. This has become important to me on many levels. To start with, when a vegetable is grown locally, it can be picked when it is ripe and sold within a few days. This means I can eat it at its most nutritious and get all the vitamins and minerals that nature meant for me to have. Usually, the fruits and vegetables you buy in the grocery store are picked well before they are ripe and then shipped across the country (or even around the globe) so that we can pretend we are supposed to be eating cherries in the middle of winter. Here's the other problem: Many of these fruits and veggies are bred over time to look stunning and endure long shipping routes, but have little taste. When I was young, I didn't even like tomatoes until I tasted one that was grown on a vine in my backyard. The ones I had tasted before were bright red, shiny and tasted like a block of wax. Yuck!

There are other, less obvious benefits to eating local foods. They can sometimes be cheaper. If you eat local foods, they are often sold when they are available by the ton and you are not paying for their plane ticket from South America. It's also better for our planet when you eat things that don't require a passport. Think of the gas we would save it we all ate just a few more locally produced foods. Finally, it's a great way to support your local economy. Here in Milwaukee I can enjoy a variety of locally farmed vegetables, ice cream and cheese made nearby from farm-fresh milk, fantastic local meats, and visit restaurants serving local foods as well.

My husband and I like to tease my mother because she always talks about how delicious the strawberries are at her grocery store. They are beautiful, big and red – but they only taste good to my mom because she covers them in artificial sweetener! I just bought fresh strawberries from a farm stand a mile from my home. They were grown less than 50 miles from where I live and their smell alone captured all that is good about summer. They tasted like heaven. No need to add sugar or artificial sweetener. Nature did that for me.

There are many ways to get local foods. Local farmers' markets can be found in almost every town these days. For people with lower incomes, many farmers' markets are now accepting food stamps. Some cities have co-ops that sell local products for a modest membership fee. Many cities publish a free flyer listing local farmers. You can start reading the addresses on food labels, and you can also talk with the manager at your grocery store to see if the store would consider carrying more local products and labeling the ones they already have. I recommend www.localharvest.org as a great resource to find a lot of information about farmers' markets, farms, stores and restaurants that have local options.

I hope that when you start to think about where your food comes from, you start to think more about what you are putting in your body. When you taste real, fresh foods, you will notice the difference for yourself.

Your Friendly Local Farmer

Community Supported Agriculture (CSA) shares are a great way to get locally grown fresh produce and to support your local economy. In a CSA, you sign up for a share or half share, which is usually delivered to a central location once a week or every other week. You pay a lump sum up front which guarantees local farmers a customer base for their produce. It also guarantees you fresh, healthy food, a closer connection to where your food is coming from, and some opportunity to sample produce you might not otherwise try. Some CSAs offer work shares, where you can work off part of the cost by helping out on the farm, or even subsidized shares for those who can't afford to pay full price.

With my local CSA, I receive an email a few days before the weekly delivery tells me what to expect and gives me the opportunity to order any specialty items such as fruits, honey, eggs, and other local products. The email also includes recipes and little notes about what was going on at the farm. The farm also schedules days for picking our own strawberries, tomatoes, and pumpkins. This gives families a true relationship with the source of where our food comes from. It encourages a respect for our land and enthusiasm for trying new foods.

What does all this local goodness cost? In our case, shares cost around $500 for the entire season of weekly deliveries from May until December. That ends up being less than $20 to $25 per week. In some areas CSAs are year-round. If not, you can make big batches of soups and store or freeze some produce for the winter months. If you can't commit to every week, there are some organizations that will allow you to buy week-to-week. To find a CSA in your area, you can visit the

Local Harvest web site I mentioned earlier. For more information on eating locally and to hear about someone's personal experience with the process, you might enjoy reading *The 100 Mile Diet*, by Alisa Smith and J.B. MacKinnon.

Organic Foods

I would love to recommend that everyone who reads this book start buying only organic foods. But here's the problem: Organic foods are more expensive. There are lots of people who really can't afford to buy organic foods. It's also important to realize that organic does not automatically mean healthy. It just means that the food or ingredients were produced without pesticides and hormones. Most people will have to make a choice about whether they can afford to buy organic foods. Luckily, there are a few resources to help.

The Environmental Working Group publishes two lists every year that can help you prioritize your organic spending and save money. The Dirty Dozen are the 12 fruits and vegetables with the most pesticide residue. These are the ones you should choose to buy organic whenever you can. The Clean Fifteen is a list of fruits and vegetables that don't require as many pesticides or that have a protective shell or peel that keeps the chemicals out of the fruit. You can find these lists in printable versions you can keep in your wallet at www.ewg.org/foodnews/summary/.

It's important to pay attention to these issues. The chemicals used to "protect" these foods from insects can cause all kinds of health problems for you. Farmers who work with pesticides often develop skin problems, breathing issues and even cancer. People who live near these farms have the same problems. Those concerns don't stop on the farm. They extend to the grocery store and to your family.

Organic fruits and vegetables may even offer more nutrition per bite. Some supporters of the organic movement say that organic produce has to work harder to maintain its own natural defenses against pests. This results in deeper root systems in healthier soil, which means more vitamins and minerals for you. These methods do require more personal attention and usually smaller farms, which is why organic food is usually more expensive. Whenever I question these price tags I remind myself that we are probably gaining a more healthy life as we grow older. These costs also keep me from buying too much junk food so there is less temptation in the house.

Under the Sea

I love seafood. Maybe you don't. (If you already think seafood is yucky, you can skip this section, although that's a shame. Fish is very good for you and comes in many flavors.) For those of you who like seafood, I have some suggestions about making good choices. As with fruits and vegetables, we need to choose the types that are less likely to be contaminated.

There are a lot of scary things floating around in our oceans, rivers and lakes. Chemicals from factories and other pollution end up in our water and then in the plants that grow in the water. The little fish eat the plants and the toxins are stored in their bodies. When bigger fish eat the little fish, the pollution really piles up. This means that it's usually better to eat the plant-eating fish instead of the fish-eating fish.

The biggest concern with seafood is mercury. Mercury builds up in big ocean fish and can cause brain damage in adults and children. Pregnant women have to be especially careful because mercury can transfer to the fetus and cause multiple birth defects.

Luckily, the Monterey Bay Aquarium created a list of the fish that are safer to eat, called Seafood Watch. They list the best fish to eat, and fish that you should eat in moderation, and the fish to avoid. The lists are divided by region in the U.S., so you will find a list specific to your area. The list is online at www.seafoodwatch.org. You can print out a little foldable sheet for your wallet or download an app to your phone so it's always with you.

What Is That Stuff?

Big Fat Fakers

I think it's great when people try to cut back on fats and sugars. I rarely hear a doctor recommend that a patient needs more fat and sugar. The problem is that we still want to eat junk foods and sweet things. This is where the scientists come in. They have been busy in the lab making chemicals that taste like food but are not. They have allowed us to pretend we are eating healthy when we are really replacing one set of problems with another.

One of my biggest concerns is artificial sweeteners. Anything that is in a box, can, jar or other container labeled "sugar-free" likely contains artificial sweeteners. There are multiple health concerns that have been associated with artificial sweeteners, but most of them need more research. One thing that has been clearly shown is that these sweeteners actually make you hungrier. The body gets all excited when it tastes the sugary flavor of the artificial sweetener and it prepares to be amazed. When it doesn't get the real deal, it's with cravings for more junk food.

Another problem with these "diet" foods is that if one thing is taken out, another thing is put in. Most "sugar-free" foods have higher carbohydrates, sodium or fat. Low-fat products often have extra sugar, which is then converted to fat by the body anyway. These foods are usually miles away from their natural form and can be hard to digest properly. They also tend to have fewer vitamins and minerals, or nutrients added back artificially. Even if you feel full after eating them, your body is left undernourished.

High-Fructose Corn Syrup

Another ingredient to avoid is high-fructose corn syrup. This seems to be in everything these days. The first problem with high-fructose corn syrup is that it is still sugar. It is not a healthy non-sugar alternative. Princeton University researchers linked this additive to increased weight gain and warning signs for diabetes. These are not side orders I want with my dinner. How about you?

Our diets are packed with corn and soy in multiple forms. Look at the ingredients in the processed foods in your pantry and you will probably find corn or soy in 80 to 90 percent of your foods. Don't get me wrong, corn and soy are good foods for you in moderation. The problem is that they are high in omega-6 fatty acids. Omega-6s are good for you in balance with omega-3s. In 2002, The National Institutes of Health recommended we should be eating only as many omega-6s as omega-3s, or a ratio of 1:1. However, thanks to all the corn and soy in our diets, the average American is consuming anywhere from 10 to 25 times as many omega-6s as omega-3s! Omega-6s are inflammatory and can lead to inflammatory diseases such as heart disease, asthma, allergies, skin conditions, arthritis, and even depression or Alzheimer's disease. To avoid this overload of omega-6s, keep an eye on processed foods and minimize your intake of fast foods. That's where the 6s are hiding out.

Looking for More Information

I hope this chapter has inspired you to pay close attention to what food you put in your body, and where your food comes from. The resources below can help you get started with healthy cooking that celebrates local ingredients.

Cookbooks

A Celebration of Wellness: A Cookbook for Vibrant Living, by James Levin, MD, and Natalie Cederquiest (Avery Publishing Group, 1992). I would buy this book just for the adorable illustrations, but it also has over 300 heart-healthy vegetarian recipes. It includes a lot of fun facts about nutrition and wellness.

Ancient Grains for Modern Meals, by Maria Speck (Ten Speed Press, 2011). This cookbook can be a little overwhelming at first because the recipes take some time to make. However, it is a great resource for learning to integrate more grains into your diet. Most people in the U.S. only eat wheat. There are so many other nutritious and tasty options available. Some health experts say that rotating the type of grains you eat is a good way to stay healthy and make sure you are getting more balance in your diet.

Bean by Bean: A Cookbook, by Crescent Dragonwagon (Workman Publishing, 2011). This cookbook reads like a story book. Plus, it's written by a woman named Crescent Dragonwagon, which is the coolest name I have ever seen. This book gives very detailed instructions for how to cook with beans, which are an excellent source of vitamins, minerals, and fiber. They are also cheap. There are recipes from all over the world in this book.

Eat to Live Cookbook: 200 Delicious Nutrient-Rich Recipes for Fast and Sustained Weight Loss, Reversing Disease, and Lifelong Health, by Joel Fuhrman (HarperOne, 2013). Dr. Fuhrman has written several books about the use of diet to reverse disease. These recipes can be challenging for people just starting to make healthy changes. The meals takes some time to make and the ingredients can be expensive. However, it focuses on nutrient-dense meals that will help you feel more energetic. (The Mushroom Stroganoff is my husband's favorite.) This is a book I recommend to friends; if you need to make immediate and significant changes due to serious illness such as heart disease or diabetes, please find it.

Food Matters: A Guide to Conscious Eating with More than 75 Recipes, by Mark Bittman (Simon & Schuster, 2009). Mark Bittman is a great writer. He starts this book with an easy-to-read explanation of why we need to change our eating habits to save our health and our planet. The second half provides menu plans and easy recipes with a lot of flexibility. Most cookbooks have exact instructions, but this one helps you learn to use local ingredients and change your cooking with the seasons.

From Asparagus to Zucchini: A Guide to Cooking Farm-Fresh Seasonal Produce, by the Madison Area Community Supported Agriculture Coalition (2004). Whether you live in the Midwest or not, this cookbook by a Wisconsin CSA coalition is a must. The book is divided by type of vegetable with some additional recipes at the end. This is the book I go to when I have a lot of one vegetable and don't know what to do with it. You can order copies at www.macsac.org.

Good and Cheap: Eat Well on $4/Day, by Leanne Brown (Workman Publishing, 2015). Leanne Brown started this book in graduate school with the idea that people could still eat healthy on $4 a day—her estimate of the average given to families on welfare. Then she took it a step further. She gave it away for FREE in an electronic format. The book has great pictures and practical recipes with clear instructions. This is a great book for people on a tight budget. Find more information at www.leannebrown.com.

Low-Fat Living Cookbook: 250 Easy, Great-Tasting Recipes, by Leslie L. Cooper (Rodale, 1998). I bought this cookbook when I was living in Dallas, more years ago than I want to admit. I had finished school, giving me more time to cook and bake, but I noticed I started gaining weight. This was one of my first healthy cookbooks, and I think I have made almost everything in this book. The recipes are easy and quick and taste great. The first part of the book offers lots of ideas for adjusting your diet to lose weight. What a treasure.

Put 'em Up!: A Comprehensive Home Preserving Guide for the Creative Cook, by Sherri Brooks Vinton (Storey, 2010). This book is so much fun! If you're interested in learning how to preserve foods using canning, drying, fermenting, freezing, etc., then this is a perfect choice. The instructions are clear, and there are many more modern and international recipes than other preserving cookbooks I have found. She includes fun ideas for making fruit-infused drinks and items with a more exotic flair.

Taste Life: Wellness Recipes for Everyday Living, from the Kanyakumari Kitchen (Blurb, 2011). Some dear friends of mine put this cookbook together. It highlights Ayurvedic recipes. Ayurveda is an ancient Indian form of medicine in which food is at the center of healing. The pictures are so beautiful in this little book. The instructions are clear, but you may have to buy some specialty items to get started. I make the Kitcheree recipe all the time—an excellent recipe to eat for a few days after you have overindulged. This cookbook can be ordered directly from Kanyakumari at www.kanyakumari.us.

The Jungle Effect, by Daphne Miller, MD (HarperCollins, 2008). I read this gem cover to cover in just a few days. Dr. Miller writes about "cold spots" in the world where certain diseases just don't seem to happen that often. She looks to the regions' diets for clues and includes lots of recipes that can help to prevent major diseases including heart disease, diabetes, prostate cancer and breast cancer. It is not technically a cookbook, but it includes much valuable information.

The Kitchen Gardener's Handbook, by Jennifer R. Bartley (Timber Press, 2010). This is a lot more than a cookbook. Jennifer Bartley includes stunning pictures, garden plans, recipes, and information on eating with the seasons. It's a beautiful and inspiring book.

The Cuisine of California, by Diane Rossen Worthington (Chronicle Books, 1997). My copy of this book is dog-eared and stained with food. I adore this book, with its focus on fresh and light ingredients. Recipes can easily be adapted to the foods you have available in your area. Try the Pesto-Stuffed Chicken Breasts or the Vegetable Frittata. We make the frittata with farm-fresh eggs. Yum!

The Gluten-Free Vegan, by Susan O'Brien (Da Capo Press, 2007). I bought this book because several of my friends are vegans and my mother-in-law is gluten-free. Most of the recipes are really easy to follow and don't take too much time. O'Brien has a Stuffed Portobello Mushroom recipe that everyone in my family loves. Living in Wisconsin, we are required to have cheese with every meal, but I make an exception for O'Brien's recipes.

The Oh She Glows Cookbook: Over 100 Vegan Recipes to Glow from the Inside Out, by Angela Liddon (Avery, 2014). This book is a current obsession. The pictures are gorgeous and Liddon has a great section about filling your pantry with staples. She also provides some delicious everyday, healthy snacks—something lacking in a lot of cookbooks. I use one of her smoothie recipes almost every day. Try the Pumpkin Pie Smoothie or The Gym Rat Smoothie. Her Nacho Dip recipe is a lifesaver for those who cannot eat dairy but wish they could. Check out free recipes at Liddon's blog www.ohsheglows.com.

The Overtown Cookbook, edited by Anthony Jennings and David Brown, MD (Booker T. Washington, 2010). This cookbook was created by a friend and former co-worker. Dr. Brown wanted to help Overtown, one of the poorest neighborhoods in Miami, by taking traditional African-American, African, and Afro-Caribbean recipes and making them healthier. He enlisted the help of the young people at Booker T. Washington High School, who took their families' recipes and transformed them in their nutrition class. I attended a cooking competition held at the high school, so I can assure you that the recipes are delicious.

Internet

www.localharvest.org
www.motherearthnews.com
www.seafoodwatch.org

Video

Mayo Clinic Wellness Solutions for Weight Loss (2008) [store.mayoclinic.com]

✓ WELL TO DO LIST
The Best Food for You

Choose one skill to practice this month, to select better food:

☐ Shop on the outside ring of the grocery store

☐ Buy things with five ingredients or less

☐ Buy things only with ingredients you recognize

☐ Buy more local foods
List where you will find these foods or ask your doctor for more information

_____

☐ Sign up for a farm share (CSA)
List which farm you will use or ask your doctor for information

_____

Circle one resource that you will look up:

The Dirty Dozen   The Clean Fifteen   Seafood Watch

Choose one cookbook or web site that provides healthy recipes, and try one new recipe a week.

List the cookbook or web site:

_____

List the recipes you have tried:

_____

_____

_____

Choose one food goal you can work toward this month:

☐ Stop drinking soda

☐ Limit soda to two times a week

☐ Stop eating at fast food restaurants

☐ Limit fast food to two times a week

☐ Reduce pre-made or boxed foods to three times a week

☐ Eat unsalted nuts instead of salty snacks

☐ Pick one day of the week to eat no meat

☐ Switch from white rice to brown rice

☐ Switch from white bread to whole-grain bread

☐ Limit dessert to three times a week

☐ Start the morning with a healthy breakfast
Please describe: _____

_____

☐ Buy or prepare healthy snacks and keep them on hand
Please describe: _____

_____

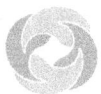

CHAPTER 5

Move It or Lose It

THERE'S A SIMPLE TREATMENT OUT THERE THAT WILL HELP YOU lose weight, improve your mood, decrease anxiety and depression, lower your blood sugar, blood pressure and cholesterol levels, make you more resistant to disease, and decrease arthritis pain. It's very reasonably priced—in fact, it's free. It's exercise! Many of my patients are taking a separate medication for each of the conditions listed above but all of them can be helped by walking for 30 minutes a day. Walking is free, easy, low impact and has very few negative side effects.

At a conference recently, I heard something downright revolutionary. The woman running the conference pointed out that we often encourage our patients to exercise by saying things like, "You might want to consider increasing your activity level," or, "It would be best if you exercise." These encouraging phrases are inadequate, she said, because we know that exercise is not "optional" or "better," it's essential. What a revelation! I no longer recommend that my patients exercise; I demand it. Our bodies are meant to move a lot throughout the day, and if they don't, they will rebel in all kinds of disturbing ways.

Most authorities on the topic are recommending 30 minutes of moderate activity most days. That may seem like a lot, but let's turn it around: I recommend that you spend 23 ½ hours relaxing each day. Does that sound better? That's what Dr. Mike Evans asks in a fun video: Can you limit your sitting and sleeping to "just 23 ½ hours" each day? Get up and walk. Dance around your house. Play with your kids or your dog. Do whatever you already like to do but just put that body in motion.

The authorities don't say that it has to be 30 minutes of *constant* activity (although that would be great). You can break it up if you need to. Take the stairs. Walk or bike to the store or to work. Walk during your lunch hour. Use a push mower instead of a rider. Wash your car by hand. Ride a stationary bike or walk on a treadmill while you watch TV. Get a pedometer and try to take 10,000 steps a day. There are so many ways to get your 30 minutes.

I have a friend who made two changes that helped him lose a lot of weight. First, he put a stationary bike in front of his TV and made himself get on it any time he watched TV. Second, whenever he received a call on his cell phone, he would take the phone outside, weather permitting, and walk around the neighborhood while he talked. Along with some modest diet changes, he was able to achieve a much healthier weight in just a few months.

The Three Musketeers: Cardio, Stretching and Strengthening

Cardio

When people start exercising, they often focus on cardiovascular (cardio) activities. These are the kinds of exercises that get your heart pumping and make you sweat. Cardio is the most effective way of burning fat and improving your heart health. As I said before, it is essential (not just "better") to get 30 minutes a day of movement, which could include walking, running, swimming, biking, dancing, martial arts, or any aerobics classes. It can also include chasing after children, gardening, taking the stairs, digging holes, cleaning the house, helping a neighbor move, or jumping up and down a lot while cheering for your favorite team. Cardio is the foundation of any good exercise plan, but there are two additional things to incorporate to ensure you have a well-rounded exercise regimen.

Stretching

Many forms of exercise cause muscles to become stiff, and high-impact exercises like running can lead to injuries and compacted tight muscles. It is important to stretch to keep muscles long and lean. There is a lot of debate about *when* and *how* to stretch. Most people now say it is best to stretch after your muscles are warm. That means that you might walk a little, stretch, and then take a run. Other people say it is best to wait until after your exercise is over. Many athletes do dynamic stretches, meaning that they do a little cardio first and then do some stretches that involve moving, such as moving lunges or forward folding and then coming back up. This is then followed by more *static* stretches like a traditional forward fold in which you hold the position.

Regardless of the exact technique, adding stretching to your exercise can help you maintain flexibility and prevent injury. Do some research or consult a personal trainer or physical therapist to help you find a safe approach.

Strengthening

No exercise program is complete without some strengthening exercises. This can include weight lifting, lunges, squats, push-ups, and abdominal work. As with cardio, this doesn't require an expensive gym membership. You can get this stuff in by gardening, cleaning, picking up the kids and carrying them, or lifting free weights while watching the latest episode of your favorite show.

Strengthening is important to build muscle mass. This form of exercise can also reduce the risk of injuries and falls, improve overall appearance, and reduce the risk of osteoporosis. Muscle also burns fat, so weight lifting can boost your weight-loss program. It's best to start a strengthening routine with a little advice from a professional—it's easy to do many of these exercises incorrectly, which can cause injuries and pain. A personal trainer, class, DVD or instructional book can get you on the right track.

Yoga: Three for the Price of One!

I think yoga is a perfect form of exercise, as it can incorporate cardio, stretching, and strengthening all at once. Some forms of yoga are intense, while others are more relaxing and may not get your heart pumping. You can easily control the intensity by which yoga you choose and how you practice it. Yoga can create long and lean muscles, decrease pain, reduce and prevent injuries, and even improve performance in sports by improving flexibility, strength and balance.

I know, you are saying to yourself that you are not a human pretzel and can't bend yourself into Cirque du Soleil postures. That's what everyone tells me. Actually, I think yoga is much better for people who are not flexible. These people really benefit from the practice, whereas super-flexible people find it too easy and often miss the mental challenge. Then there are the men who say yoga is for women, to which I respond that LeBron James does yoga. Enough said.

There are hundreds of different kinds of yoga. It may take some time to find the kind that you like best. If you like high-energy classes that keep moving and are physically challenging, you should try Power Yoga or Vinyasa Flow. If you like to master things and enjoy doing the same routine regularly, you may want to look for an Ashtanga class. This is a set series that you can learn and then do on your own at home. If you are detail-oriented or have injuries you are concerned about, Iyengar yoga is probably best for you. These instructors are well trained in modifying poses using props and adjustments that can actually resolve injuries over time. Another option for those with injuries or specific concerns or goals is Yoga Therapy. Most yoga therapists receive 1,000 hours or more of training in the therapeutic benefits of the poses. If you need to relax from your busy life, you may want to try restorative or gentle yoga classes. If you are pregnant, it's usually best to find a prenatal yoga class in your area to ensure that you are doing poses that are safe for pregnant women. Plus, it's fun to practice with other future moms.

If you want to learn the basics, you can start with a Hatha yoga class or a beginners class. Many yoga studios offer a series of four to six classes for beginners to learn the basics.

Yoga type	Best for	Description

Power Yoga or Vinyasa Flow	Lots of movement	High-energy classes that keep moving and are physically challenging.
Ashtanga	Mastering a set series	A set series that you can learn and then do on your own at home. Features increasing difficulty as you practice longer.
Iyengar Yoga	Those who are injured or naturally cautious	Instructors are well trained in modifying poses using props and adjustments that can actually resolve injuries over time.
Yoga Therapy	Special requirements	Helpful if you are injured or have other special requirements, with a focus on the therapeutic benefits of the poses.
Gentle Yoga or Restorative Yoga	Relaxing, recovering	An opportunity to relax from your busy life.
Hatha Yoga or Beginner Yoga	Learning the basics	A good foundation in yoga principles and poses.
Prenatal Yoga	Pregnancy	Yoga classes specially designed for the needs during pregnancy.

Be sure to read class descriptions ahead of time and don't be afraid to call and ask questions. I also recommend talking to the instructor before class to say that you are new or that you have a particular injury or health concern.

While there are great yoga videos, I recommend trying yoga first with an instructor and then trying it at home. Instructors can help you learn how to get into poses safely, and answer any questions that come up as you try new ones. Most of us have no idea how out of alignment our bodies have become over time. When I teach yoga, I often say, "Roll your shoulders away from your ears," only to watch those shoulders creep back up again. Maybe you just had to lower yours now. There are also people who are double-jointed and don't realize it. This can cause strain on muscles and joints and cause injuries over time if not corrected.

The Right Tool for the Job

Joining a gym can be fun but can also be expensive. With a small investment of a few tools, you can have an effective gym at home. I recommend starting with a few stretchy bands in different levels of resistance, a set of light weights (three to five pounds) and a set of more heavy weights (eight to 10 pounds). Adding an exercise/yoga mat and exercise ball will make core strengthening more comfortable. If you have a little extra cash to invest, there are lots of used treadmills and stationary bikes for sale online and at garage sales. We found a treadmill for less than $250 and have used it every week for six years! If you have the discipline, there are a few DVDs I recommend that are fun and will save you money if you use them over a period of time.

Cardio

Try Zumba videos if you like music and dancing. These videos are a lot of fun, but they can be difficult to follow for some people and they are high-impact, meaning they are not a good place to start if you have chronic pain or are a beginner. These videos are sold in packages so they can be a little expensive. They can be found at www.zumba.com.

If you are a beginner, older, or need something less rump-shaking than Zumba, one of the best video series I have found is Leslie Sansone's *Walk at Home* series. It's low-impact, super easy to follow, and most of the videos come with choices depending on how much time you have on a particular day. That means you are getting several workouts for the price of one. Her videos can be found at www.walkathome.com. My mother is in great shape, and she credits these videos.

Yoga

As I described above, yoga is a great way to exercise and form long, lean muscles. It has numerous health benefits and is a great choice for cross-training for almost any sport. Many runners and athletes benefit from the injury prevention offered by yoga. You can find great free yoga videos at www.doyogawithme.com.

If you like DVDs, I can recommend the 2008 DVD set *Yoga for Beginners and Beyond* by bodywisdom media. This set reviews the foundations of yoga, has several practices to choose from, and even includes a special practice for people who feel they cannot do yoga because they are too stiff and inflexible. It's reasonably priced for the amount of material included. Rodney Yee is another great instructor for beginners. He is well respected in the field, offers clear instruction, and has videos available for any level or need at www.gaiam.com/yoga-videos/. Pregnant women will enjoy Anna

Getty's *Pre and Post Natal Yoga Workout,* or Sara Holliday's *Prenatal Yoga* Series, which is a set of three DVDs divided by trimester. There are many options to get you started, so give it a try and you may change your life.

Core Strength

If you want to work on your core strength and abdominal muscles, you should try Pilates. This is a method of exercises that targets the abdomen, thighs and buttocks (who couldn't use a little help there?). The exercises range from easy to extremely difficult. It's very important to watch your alignment when doing Pilates. Improper alignment can lead to neck, shoulder, and back pain. I recommend Mari Winsor's videos. She provides clear instructions and lots of modifications if you are just starting. Her collection can be found at www.winsorpilates.com.

Personal trainer Gunnar Peterson has made several excellent videos that focus on core strengthening. He gives good cues, safe modifications for beginners, and doesn't add a lot of silly commentary. Most of his videos have choices to modify the workout depending on how late you slept in that day. He often incorporates weights and the exercise ball, and you are so distracted by trying not to fall off the darned thing that you don't even notice you are working out. One of his newest releases is *Shape: Best- Ever Hollywood Workout.*

The Best Things in Life Are Free

Exercise does not have to cost anything, even with instruction. There are a lot of YouTube videos, podcasts, and web sites that offer free workouts. Your local library will also carry workout videos. Many cable services offer free on-demand workouts and most public television stations have regular exercise shows. Many hospital libraries have a huge collection of videos. Check out used bookstores or thrift stores for great values on workout DVDs. You may find some really bad ones, but there are likely some treasures as well.

Do What You Love

As I mentioned at the beginning of this chapter, exercise may improve your immunity. This means exercise helps keep you from getting sick—but there's a catch. Newer research shows that this is only true *if you like the exercise you are doing*. If you choose a form of exercise you hate, it can actually reduce your resistance to disease, meaning that you are more likely to get sick. This is why I personally avoid things like running and super high-impact aerobics, which some other people love.

The trick to a lifelong exercise routine that is to find one that is fun to do—for you. Some people may love to do the same thing for years, while others need to make sure the routine is always changing. I keep a library of exercise DVDs in my basement and I organize them so that every day I am doing something new. This keeps my body challenged and my mind interested. It also keeps me from trying to decide which video to do when I am tired and feeling lazy. I just have to do whatever video is next in line. I don't always work out alone. I sign up for classes with friends and I take group classes at a local gym that involve loud pop music—they make me feel like I'm in a music video.

You probably have a different idea of a good time than I do. Give yourself a chance to figure out what works for you and leaves you feeling happy and energized. You may not be excited when you *start* a workout, but notice which workout makes you feel good when you are done. Try out different ideas and see which activities help you forget you are exercising. Whatever you choose, just keep doing it. If it stops being fun, find something else, but never stop moving. Move like your life depends on it, because it does.

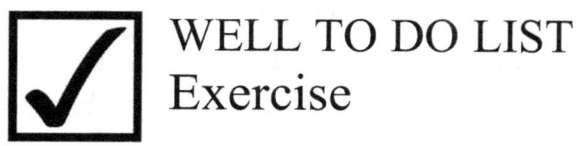

WELL TO DO LIST
Exercise

Look at your calendar. Every week for the next 4 weeks, find three days where you can do 30 minutes of movement and schedule it in like an appointment.

List the Exercise Appointments:

Week	Day/Time	Day/Time	Day/Time
1			
2			
3			
4			

What kind of movement will you do? _____

_____

Which activity timing will you do on each scheduled day? *(Circle one)*

    30 min   2x15 min   3x10 min

List one cardio_activity you do or could do. *(Consult with your doctor for safety.)*

_____   _____   _____

Activity   Frequency   Duration

List one area of your body that you need to stretch more often:

_____

List one stretch you can do daily for the next week that will address the area listed above. *(Consult with your doctor for safety.)*

_____	_____	_____
Activity	Frequency	Duration

List one strengthening activity you do or could do. *(Consult with your doctor for safety.)*

_____	_____	_____
Activity	Frequency	Duration

List one video, product or piece of equipment you can invest in in the next month that will increase your movement:

_____

CHAPTER 6

Breathe Easy - Stop Smoking

IF YOU ARE A SMOKER, I HOPE YOU ARE READING THIS CHAPTER because it means that you have at least considered becoming smoke-free. Great idea! I vote yes! If you are really ready, congratulations on your decision to stop smoking! Your physician is eager to help you through the process of regaining your health, independence and freedom. Below, you will find some concrete skills that will help you set goals and measure your success along the way.

I'm sure you already know that smoking is really bad for you. Horrible, in fact. Smoking can affect everything from your ability to breathe well to your ability to digest food properly. It irritates allergies and asthma, and increases your likelihood of catching colds and other viruses. Smoking increases the risk of heart attacks and can cause problems with sleep. It causes headaches and can even affect your memory and ability to concentrate. In general, it keeps the body from healing itself the way it is designed to.

Smoking also causes major problems for the people around you. This is an especially big problem if you are around children. Second-hand smoke increases the number of ear infections and respiratory infections in children. It increases their chances of getting asthma, and can even increase the risk of Sudden Infant Death Syndrome (SIDS). Even the small amount of tobacco left on your clothes, hair and skin puts other people at risk. You may already know all of this.

The good news is that many of the health problems caused by smoking can begin to reverse themselves right away. When you stop smoking, your body will immediately start to heal and your heart and lungs will improve within days. Some researchers even think that within a few years you will be almost as healthy as people who never smoked. What are you waiting for? If you are reading this, hopefully you are ready to **make a plan** and **take action**.

First Steps

You may feel like this is a decision that you will have to ease your way into. Not everyone can or should stop smoking "cold turkey." There are several things you can do to prepare yourself before you actually stop smoking.

Switch Brands

There are so many images out there telling us that smoking is manly, sexy, exotic or cool. Think about images such as the Marlboro man. This image would have you believe that smoking will make you tough and that you might be able to herd cattle if you would only smoke these cigarettes. For years, professional women's tennis was sponsored by Virginia Slims cigarettes. I find that especially ironic considering how hard it is to play tennis well when you are a smoker. Virginia Slims also has many advertisements featuring thin, elegant women.

All of these images make an impression. Over time, you start to believe that a certain brand makes you a certain kind of person. Smoking can often be very tied into that image. Shaking that image a bit can be the first step toward shaking the hold that smoking may have on you.

Try switching brands for a few days and see how you feel. Some of my clients are surprised at how hard this is to do. It makes them realize how much they are influenced by marketing. Others notice that they feel physically different, even ill. This reminds many people how much of a physical influence tobacco has on the body and how processed and unnatural these tobacco products are.

As a side note, it might be interesting for you to know that all of the men who modeled as the Marlboro Man have died of lung cancer. Is that the image that you want to follow?

Learn to Breathe for Relaxation

Most people who ask me for help to stop smoking say that it is the only thing that helps them relax and manage stress. That sounds funny, because nicotine is actually a stimulant. It makes us feel anxious, tense, and sometimes irritable. The tricky thing about nicotine is that it takes a while to kick in.

What does everyone tell you when you need to relax? They usually say something like, "Take a deep breath." What do you do when you are smoking? You take deep breaths. You also usually have to step away, often go outside. So, in order to smoke, you walk away from your normal surroundings and then take some time to breathe deeply.

I would argue that it's this combination of movement, separation, and deep breathing that help you relax and change your mood. Then, just as you are feeling good, you return to work, or life in general, and the nicotine kicks in and makes you feel anxious. You mistakenly think that it is returning to the environment that causes all the stress.

I'm not saying that life is only stressful because you use nicotine, but I do want to point out that you undo all the benefits of that great stress management routine (walking away, being outdoors, inhaling deeply) by using a stimulant that is known to cause anxiety! Then you keep using it hoping that it's helping you cope with stress when it actually makes things much worse. A "smoke break" is the perfect stress reliever, if you remove the cigarette from the process. My suggestion is to take breathing breaks instead of smoke breaks. Throughout the day, get in the habit of stepping away from what you are doing, getting outside if possible, and breathing deeply. Notice whether the benefits of these practices last longer without the nicotine.

Identify Triggers

Do you only smoke when you are drinking alcohol? Always smoke in the car on your drive to work? Maybe you smoke when you are bored or right after you eat. Maybe you only smoke on days ending in Y. Most people will tell you that there are things that signal them to smoke. These are your *triggers,* and may include things like stress, time of day, particular people, or avoiding conflict.

What comes to mind for you? Can you point to certain times or situations that lead you to smoke or to smoke more? If you want to stop smoking, then you will need to take some time to think about these triggers. You will also need to start making a plan to avoid these triggers.

Avoiding triggers can be a difficult process for many people because it often means avoiding favorite places and people until you no longer have the urge to smoke. This is easier now because many states have indoor smoking bans that make it difficult for people to smoke in most public places. In some cases, these laws even extend to outdoor locations.

Finding Replacement Activities

In addition to avoiding triggers, you can look for some replacement behaviors that help take the place of smoking.

Oral Fixation

Carl came to me with a real desire to stop smoking. When we talked about triggers, he was able to identify that he spends a lot of time in the car because he works in sales. He gets bored and fidgety in the car. In fact, he said that he chewed on pens in school all the time. He felt that he has always needed something to chew on or in his mouth when he's sitting still. He came up with the idea of having a bag of straws in the car to chew. This really helped him, but did leave a long trail of massacred straws. Others have used chewing gum and hard candy to accomplish the same goal.

You will want to be careful not to trade cavities and calories for smoking by overdoing the sweets. Sugar-free gum is a good option—it's inexpensive and easy to buy everywhere. I'm not usually a fan of artificial sweeteners, but if it can help you to stop smoking, it's a big step in the right direction.

Keeping Hands Busy

When I was living in Miami, a doctor asked me to join her with her patient for a consultation to stop smoking. I entered the room to find a very dignified and handsome older Cuban gentleman. He wanted desperately to stop smoking so that he could see his grandchildren grow up. After talking to him for a few minutes we figured out that he started smoking to have something to do with his hands.

Have you ever seen *Top Gun*? There's a scene in that movie where Val Kilmer's "Ice Man" twirls a pen all along his fingers during a briefing. If you've ever tried it you know that it's really hard to do. I taught our patient how to do this as best I could, and he smiled so brightly that it lit up the room. I gave him my pen and asked him to take good care of it. His doctor prescribed him a nicotine patch and we asked him to report back in a month.

The next month he was smoke-free and an expert pen twirler. He bragged that he was now teaching his grandchildren to do this. He still had my pen.

Avoidance

Some people smoke when they are upset. It gives them an excuse to get out of the house or office and avoid dealing with the problem directly. It may take some time to learn how to talk calmly about conflicts and to resolve them peacefully. In this case, a counselor can be really helpful in teaching you techniques for resolving underlying problems directly. They are really easy once you learn them. Take a look at Chapter 9 on Stress Management for some ideas to get you started.

Nicotine Replacement

The nicotine in cigarettes is a powerful addictive drug, and there are many symptoms associated with nicotine withdrawal including anger, irritability, anxiety, cravings, decreased concentration, hunger, weight gain, restlessness, drowsiness, fatigue, impaired task performance, and sleep disturbance. You may also struggle with some physical reactions. Some people stop smoking and never feel a thing, but most people experience feelings ranging from uncomfortable to miserable.

The good news is that you can get help avoiding these symptoms. There are many products on the market that can help you through the first few weeks or months smoke -free. Nicotine patches, gums, and lozenges may be just the thing for you. Others switch to electronic cigarettes or e-cigarettes, which are tobacco-free but still deliver nicotine. (Remember that the safety of these e-cigs, for smokers and bystanders, is still in question.) There are also medications that can be helpful. All medications should be discussed with your doctor. Some of these medications can interact with other medications you might be taking and can be dangerous.

Nagging Means I Love You

Many people tell me they find it really annoying and frustrating when their friends and family "nag them all the time" to stop smoking. I get it, but to be honest, if one of my family members were smoking, I would do the same thing. This kind of nagging often makes people dig in their heels about smoking. The smoker may think, "If I stop smoking, then I'm admitting that the people who have been nagging me are right, and I was wrong." No one wants to be wrong. Or maybe you just don't like to be told what to do, or feel attacked and judged by those who tell you to stop smoking.

I encourage smokers to try to think about this "nagging" in a different way. Remind yourself that when someone you love encourages you to stop smoking he or she is really saying, **"I love you and would like to keep you around for a long time."** A friend may be saying, "I like to spend time with you, but I fear for my own health or the health of my children due to second-hand smoke." Either way, it means someone cares and would like to be with you longer and more often. I sure hope there are few people who feel that way about me. Don't you?

Ready, Set, Go!

I hope you're ready to take the next step and stop smoking. The following section may give you some ideas for how to get started and stay smoke-free.

Quitters Never Win

Have you noticed that this is the first time I have used the word "quit" in this chapter? I like to call this "the Q word." The thing is, in our society quitting has a really negative sound to it. No one wants to be a quitter. I've noticed that many stop smoking campaigns sponsored by the tobacco companies (because they are forced to do it) use the Q word. Other stop smoking initiatives use more positive phrases like "Get the truth."

I have stopped encouraging people to "quit" and have started asking them to "stop smoking." It's a small change, but one that I think can really make a difference in your attitude toward the whole idea.

If You Knew Then What You Know Now

My grandfather started smoking at 12 years old and, despite warnings from many doctors, he kept smoking until he died. He would hide in his car and smoke. After he died, we found packs of cigarettes hidden in plant pots and under the car seat. His doctors told him that he would die if he kept smoking, and even then he could not stop. I often wonder, if he had known in the beginning how much damage it would do, would he have started in the first place?

I have asked many people this question, and I still have not met anyone would have started smoking if he or she had known how hard it would be to stop or how much damage it would do to their bodies and their relationships. When was the last time you had a cigarette? Maybe it was two minutes ago or maybe it was two hours ago. You can choose to start to live smoke-free right now, or at any time.

Breathing Skills/Adult Time Out

As I mentioned before, one of the reasons you feel so relaxed after a cigarette is because you are practicing deep breathing. You can do that without a cigarette. Even taking five deep belly breaths can help you to relax and manage stress. It is even better if you can remove yourself physically from a situation that is causing stress.

I have a young child, and we are using a lot of *time outs* at the moment. The idea behind time outs is not punishment so much as a time for kids to remove themselves from a stressful situation and calm down a bit before trying to resolve a conflict. That seems like something adults should do as well. Actually, I think adults need time outs more than kids do.

I have met a lot of mothers who tell me that they can't get away from the chaos. I sometimes recommend that they lock themselves in the bathroom for a few minutes and try to tune out the noise and breathe for a bit before trying to control whatever craziness is happening in the rest of the house. You can also use a bike ride, a walk, or reading the paper as a time out. The idea is that when you feel you are about to lose control, you separate yourself physically or mentally from stress before you try to resolve it.

Light a Candle

Every time I go camping, I spend the first hour wondering what the heck we'll do to stay entertained for the whole time. By the time night rolls around, I find that I could stare at the campfire for hours. It's better than TV. A safe, contained fire is very hypnotic.

Smoking has all kinds of hypnotic things associated with it. First you light a fire, then you take a deep breath, and then the smoke twirls calmly into the air. There are healthy ways to duplicate this feeling. I learned to do Candle Meditation when I was taking a Kung Fu class a few years ago. It is very relaxing and can help focus your thoughts and teach you to calm your mind without cigarettes. It is also very easy to do.

There are two ways to do this meditation. The first is to stare at a candle and try to move the flame with your thoughts. The alternative way to do this is to stare at the candle and try to keep the flame still. I like this version because I think it encourages me to be very still and to breathe slowly and gently. Obviously this isn't something that most people can do at work, but it is something that can be integrated into a daily relaxation practice.

Pay the Piper

Sometimes when trying to stop a bad habit, people put money in a jar every time they do the offending behavior. They may donate the money to a charity. The problem with this idea is that you could tell yourself that you are now "smoking for a cause." I suggest you can flip this around, to start collecting money for a group you don't like very much.

One of my patients was a staunch Republican, so he started collecting money for the Democratic Party. Another patient of mine hated guns, so he collected for the National Rifle Association. One of my girlfriends used to make her husband put $5 towards her "purse fund" every time he smoked—she got a fancy Coach purse out of it before he quit. The point is to suffer a little bit every time you have to pay up. Obviously this will only work if you are a very honest person and will actually follow through. If you need a little help getting started check out www.stickk.com.

Do Yoga

I'm a yoga evangelist because yoga is beneficial for so many problems. It helps different people in different ways. If you are learning to live smoke-free, yoga can help you learn to breathe again. It can undo the tension built up from years of nicotine use. Yoga helps you be more aware of your body and identify stress and manage it. This may prevent the need for a cigarette. Yoga can even help you learn breathing skills that keep you calm enough to deal properly with the conflicts you used to avoid by taking a smoke break. Finally, yoga can help you avoid weight gain that people often experience after they stop smoking.

Relapse

Some people stop smoking and tell me that they never miss it. I admire these people, but I think most people need to stop a few times before it becomes permanent. In fact, the average person needs to stop smoking four to eight times before it sticks. I say, let's get started! Maybe you can stop smoking four times today and get it all out of the way. But even if you do stop smoking, you might have a small setback from time to time.

Try to think of one cigarette as a mistake rather than an excuse to chuck the whole idea and start smoking again. The best way to deal with relapse is first to realize that it may happen. The second step is to have a plan for how you will deal with it. My suggestion is to plan to forgive yourself quickly and get back to work. Again, identifying your triggers will help you to avoid the problem altogether, but if you do slip up, just acknowledge the error, look at the ideas above, figure out what went wrong, and fix it so it doesn't happen again.

Be Amazing

I believe that everyone has the potential to be amazing. But the truth is that tobacco will drain you of the energy or motivation to be everything you are capable of. Both you and the world deserve to see the best you have to offer.

In the time you just spent between now and your last cigarette, you stopped smoking. Congratulations, you're already off to a great start!

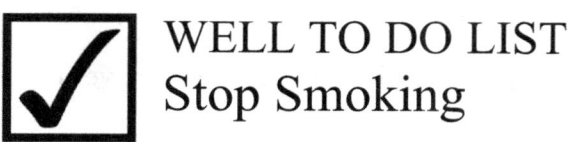

WELL TO DO LIST
Stop Smoking

How is smoking working for you?

_____

What do you not like about smoking?

_____

_____

First Steps: Choose one strategy below you can use for the next month, and answer the question about that strategy.

☐ Switch brands
Which brand will you use?

☐ Do yoga
Where and when will you attend?

☐ Practice taking "breathing breaks"
What time will you do this?

☐ Candle Meditation
What time will you do this?

☐ Avoid triggers
List one trigger you will avoid.

☐ Find a replacement activity
List a replacement activity.

☐ Pay the Piper
How much will you pay? What charity will you support? Who will monitor this?

☐ Adult time outs/Breathing skills
Where will you go and which specific breathing skill will you use?

What is most likely to cause a relapse?

_____

_____

How will you handle a relapse and get back on track?

_____

_____

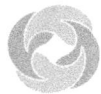

CHAPTER 7

Rest Is Best

Early to bed and early to rise, makes a man healthy, wealthy and wise.

—Benjamin Franklin

I MET "FRANK" LAST MONTH WHILE WORKING IN THE HOSPITAL. He was in our rehabilitation unit struggling with some physical limitations after a cancer-related surgery. Frank had been given steroids, which make it very hard to sleep well, and he was totally exhausted. He was also irritable and short-tempered, which his wife said was unusual for him.

Frank told me that he had been able to fall asleep, but the hospital staff were waking him up every two hours throughout the night for various reasons. I talked with his nurse to see if there was any reason he would absolutely have to be awakened during the night. We could not find anything that would require disturbing our patient's sleep.

We posted a sign on the door that day stating, "Please do not disturb between 10 p.m. and 6 a.m.," and it worked perfectly. Frank was able to sleep for five hours the next night and even longer the following night. On our next visit, his mood was drastically improved. He was making jokes and telling me how much he appreciated the care he was receiving. What a difference a good night of sleep can make!

Sleep Is Essential

Sleep is essential to health and well-being. It's the body's time to recharge, and the brain's time to solidify learning, store memories and solve problems. It disappoints me that we have to post signs on a patient's door to remind healthcare professionals that a person who is ill needs a good night's sleep.

What disappoints me even more is how much we deprive ourselves of sleep. Between 12 and 15 percent of Americans have serious sleep problems, with another 20 to 25 percent complaining of trouble sleeping some of the time. According to the National Institutes of Health (NIH), about 60 million Americans experience insomnia on a regular basis and many more suffer from problems such as nightmares, sleepwalking and health conditions that keep them from getting a good night's sleep.

As you get older, you spend less time in bed. As a baby, you can spend up to 17 hours a day sleeping. At the age of 12 you need about 10 hours of sleep and between the ages of 25 and 45 this lowers to about 7 ½ hours. After 45, there is a return to 8 ½ hours spent in bed, but less time is spent actually sleeping. In later years, the average sleep time is around 6 ½ hours. Also, sleep for older people becomes choppier, as they wake up more and more often and have a hard time getting back to sleep. This is caused by decreasing levels of a chemical called melatonin in the brain and body.

Age Group	Recommended Hours of Sleep
Infant	14 to 15 hours
Toddler	12 to 14 hours
School-Age Children	10 to 11 hours
Adults	7 to 9 hours

Recommended Hours of Sleep by Age Group

How Lack of Sleep Affects Your Life

Getting enough sleep doesn't just make you feel better. It is actually *required* for a healthy and happy life. Some patients tell me that they only need a few hours of sleep a night to function, but research consistently shows that people with more than seven hours of sleep perform better on mental tasks than those who get less sleep. Here is what you can become when you don't get enough sleep:

Cranky	Mood is one of the first things to be changed by sleep loss. With even a little sleep loss, our ability to deal with anger and frustration is much lower. This can cause problems with friends, family, and workmates.
Overwhelmed	Lack of sleep may lead to very strong feelings of not being able to handle even simple problems. You will worry more and be more nervous and frustrated. You may also overreact to small problems in your life.

Withdrawn	Because you feel so tired, you may begin to avoid interacting with other people because it just takes too much energy. Have you ever found yourself wishing you had not made plans for a Friday night because it just seems like too much effort to go out?
Overweight	People often eat and drink foods high in sugar in order to stay awake for some activity. Others use food to comfort stress and boredom that may be caused by lack of sleep. Also, lack of sleep releases stress hormones that can cause the body to store fat.
Sick	The body's natural methods of fighting disease may slow down or even stop working if a person has not had enough sleep. This means that you are more likely to get sick when you sleep less.
Unproductive	The brain works more slowly and reaction times increase. Creativity, logic, decision-making and coordination are also affected by lack of sleep.

The Well-Rested Person

Often we don't even realize how affected we are by a lack of sleep because we are used to working and living with lower levels of alertness. Many of us have been sleepy for such a long time that we don't know what it is like to feel totally awake and rested. When you are well-rested, you:

- Wake up naturally and without an alarm at the time that you need to get up.
- Remain energetic throughout the day, with a small dip in energy in the afternoon that might require a short nap or rest period.
- Are able to complete your chores and activities without feeling burdened or overwhelmed.
- Are able to stay awake when sitting still, such as when you are reading.
- Are able to perform mentally demanding tasks to the best of your ability.
- Feel tired (not exhausted) but calm when it is time to go to sleep.

Ideas for a Better Night's Sleep

The following steps provide a recipe for healthy sleep habits. We tend to break these rules when we are under stress or overly busy. Adding some simple stress and time management skills to your daily routine will also improve your sleep. Remember that the more stressed you are, the more you need a good night of sleep to help you face this stress. Following these suggestions may help. Managing your daytime stress will help even more (see Chapter 9).

Give It Time

Sleep as much as you need to feel refreshed and healthy the next day but no more. Limiting the time in bed seems to make people sleep better when they are in bed. Spending a very long time in bed can lead to choppy and light sleep. When you are experiencing a lot of stress, it is even more important to keep a regular sleep schedule.

Get on a Schedule

It's best to go to sleep and get up at the same time every day. The body runs on cycles and doing the same thing every day lets your body know when it is time to be awake and time to be sleepy. I know this one sounds impossible. However, I did this for one full year in graduate school and it made a huge difference in my school performance and my mood.

Exercise

Exercising *regularly* can lead to deeper sleep over time. However, exercising one time will not help you to sleep better the following night.

Quiet Time

Loud noises can disturb sleep even when you don't remember waking. Try to keep your bedroom as quiet as possible.

Climate Control

Although some people prefer to sleep in a cold room, there is no proof that this leads to better sleep. Try to find ways to make the temperature comfortable for you. Wear the amount of clothing you need to stay cool or warm and have an extra blanket ready on cold nights.

Snacks

A small snack before bed may help. Warm milk contains chemicals that can actually help you relax and may help you sleep. Keep in mind, this does not mean you should eat a lot right before bed, as that can cause acid reflux (heartburn) and also keep you awake.

Keep It Natural

Sleeping pills can help on rare occasions, but if used regularly they can actually interfere with sleep and can cause health problems.

Caffeine

Caffeine can stay in your body for six to eight hours. Caffeinated drinks such as soda and coffee are very likely to disrupt sleep even in people who don't notice the effects. They are likely to keep you up later than is necessary, which will result in feeling tired the next day, which will cause you to drink more caffeine to feel alert. If you struggle with sleep, it may be best to cut out all caffeine, or, if that's too challenging, avoid caffeine after noon.

Watch the Cocktails

Alcohol can help a tense person fall asleep, but that person is then more likely to have a poor night's sleep and may be unable to get back to sleep when the effects of the alcohol wear off.

Stop Smoking

Pretty please! Nicotine energizes you just like caffeine. Smoking increases blood pressure and pulse, which can also disturb sleep.

Bath Time

Take a warm bath or shower before bed. This will help you to feel relaxed and tired. Also it will raise your body temperature. As your body temperature begins to lower again, it will cause you to feel sleepy.

Routine

Try to do the same things, in the same order, every night before you go to bed. As this becomes habit, it will trigger your body and mind to feel sleepy. Reading, having a cup of tea, meditation, prayer, walking the dog, brushing your teeth, and even making lunches and laying out clothes for the next day can all be rituals that signal the body and mind that rest is coming soon.

Timing

Instead of trying harder and harder to get to sleep on a rough night, turn on the light and do something else for a while. Return to bed when you feel tired again.

Just Say "No" to TV

Get that TV out of your bedroom. In fact, you should avoid any exposure to screens that light up, such as smartphones, tablets and laptop monitors, for the hour before you go to bed. These lights confuse the body into thinking it is light outside. Your brain then sends out chemicals that cause you to feel more awake. If you cannot possibly bear to part with your computer before bed, you might try f.lux, a program that adjusts your screen's lighting depending on the time of day. Find more information on this free (at press time) download at justgetflux.com.

Take a News Break

While we're talking about TV, you may want to consider a break from the news in the evening. If you really struggle with stress, you may want to take a longer break and consider avoiding news for a few weeks until you sleep better. Studies have linked the type of news shown on most networks with increased rates of depression. Andrew Weil, MD, recommends a "News Fast" as one of 10 Simple Ways to Improve Your Health.

Relax

Use relaxation techniques such as breathing slowly or relaxing tense muscles in order to calm down before going to sleep. I'll describe how to do some of these techniques in detail, and you may be surprised at how easy and effective they can be.

Relaxation Exercises

As noted above, one of the best ways to ensure a good night of rest is to begin sleep in a relaxed state. There are several relaxation exercises that can easily be done in a resting position. Use the following Skill Prescription exercises to relax and get ready for sleep.

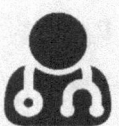

Skill Prescription:

Relaxation Exercises

Progressive Muscle Relaxation (PMR)

Try tensing and then relaxing your muscles in groups, starting from the toes and slowly working up the body to the eye muscles and forehead. Squeeze tightly for five to 10 seconds, then release and relax for 15 to 20 seconds before moving up to the next group of muscles. *See the Stress Management Chapter for more details on PMR.*

Mattress Yoga

Begin lying on your bed with your arms at your sides. Relax and inhale to the count of five, and while breathing raise your arms up and back over your head until they touch the mattress. Make two fists and raise your lower back off the mattress. Tense and stretch every muscle, even your face. Then, arms still raised, let all the tension drain from your body.

Visualization

Imagine yourself in a relaxing place such as lying on a tropical beach, walking in a field, floating in the air, or listening to soft music. Feel the warmth of the sun and the gentle breezes, hear the waves, and smell the air. Relax.

Deep Breathing

Take five deep breaths, and as you count each one, say to yourself, "I'm getting more relaxed, peaceful, and quiet. I'm slowly falling asleep." Concentrate only on this message.

Mind Games

Imagine you are writing huge numbers on a long blackboard. Start at 100 and work your way back to one. My grandmother used to tell me to imagine a blackboard full of my concerns and worries from the day, then imagine erasing each word or phrase one by one until the board is blank.

How to Avoid the Morning Slump

How you get up in the morning can influence your entire day. Start off the morning in a grumpy, irritable mood and the rest of the day probably will not go well. Start off the day feeling good and the rest of your day will probably go much better.

You may be starting your mornings off on the wrong foot if you hit the snooze button and tell yourself that you can rush and get ready in 30 minutes instead of the usual hour. This extra 30 minutes of sleep will probably not make you feel more rested. You will not really fall asleep, but instead will enter a kind of mental state between asleep and awake. When you finally do get up, you will not feel as rested as you would have if you had just gotten up when the alarm first sounded. Also, by giving yourself less time to get ready, you are now starting the day with added stress that may affect the rest of the day. By getting up right away from the sleep state and starting a normal morning routine you may have a more positive attitude towards yourself and your day.

Morning activities such as walking the dog, reading the newspaper, or packing a lunch for the kids or yourself help you begin the day by accomplishing goals. The sooner you become physically and mentally active, the more you will feel able to face the day feeling alert and confident. On the other hand, if the morning routine is actually causing stress, you may want to consider laying out your clothes and packing up lunches the night before so that you can start your day with more time and less stress.

Is It Naptime Yet?

Napping is a lost art in our modern culture. It's often seen as an act of laziness, but many very successful people in history thought of naps as a way to maximize their day and to stay alert and sharp all day. Winston Churchill is said to have arranged all his cabinet meetings around his nap schedule.

Research shows that the human body has a natural need to rest in the middle of the afternoon. This is needed even after a good night of sleep. Our body temperature drops quite a bit at night and makes us tired, but it also drops a bit in the middle of the day. This usually happens 12 hours after the middle of our night's rest. This means that most people will feel a slump between 2 p.m. and 4 p.m.

There are several benefits to getting a daily nap, including the following:

- **Less Stress**: A study showed that people in countries that have a siesta are less stressed than North Americans.
- **Healthy Heart**: The risk of heart disease may be reduced by a 30-minute daily nap.
- **Better Focus**: Naps help to improve the ability to pay attention to details and make important decisions.

- **Time Out**: Naps taken about eight hours after you wake have been shown to do much more for you than if you just added 20 minutes to the amount of time spent sleeping during the night.

The Power Nap

Not everyone has time for the recommended 20 to 40 minutes a real nap requires, and unfortunately most of our employers would frown on napping on the job (although they shouldn't). Another option is the five- to 10-minute seated power nap. The famous painter Salvador Dali took naps seated and holding a spoon above a plate set on the floor. As soon as he fell asleep, the spoon would hit the plate and wake him up. He claimed he just needed to fall asleep to feel rested. Interestingly, he would then immediately record what he had seen in his dreamlike state and this helped him generate ideas for his paintings.

I like to think of a power nap as an opportunity to "reboot" the mind. Some people claim that a short nap of five to 10 minutes has a refreshing result by clearing the mind of past activities, reducing tension and increasing energy to complete a new task. Each person has a specific period of time needed to achieve this effect. For some, five minutes is all that is needed. Others need a bit more. However, if you spend too much time napping (more than 40 minutes), then you will enter a true sleep state and when you wake up you will feel negative effects such as confusion, tiredness, and irritability.

The following Skill Prescription provides some tips on how to take a "power nap" or a short nap to feel refreshed and energized.

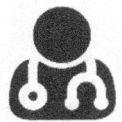

Skill Prescription:

Take a Power Nap

1. Set an alarm if you need to. (Hint, most cell phones can do a timer or alarm).
2. Find a comfortable position, but not one that will allow you to sleep deeply. This is not the time to go to bed. Use any of the relaxation skills presented in this chapter to quiet yourself.
3. Try to quiet your mind and slow down your thoughts. Thinking of a peaceful and relaxing place such as a beach may help.
4. Relax your eyes and allow them to close gently.
5. If you usually fall asleep easily, put yourself in a less comfortable position, such as sitting up in a chair, so that you will have to remain somewhat alert in order to stay in the position.
6. Start by experimenting with a five- to 10-minute session. If you don't feel refreshed, you can extend the time period.

Renewing Energy

Sometimes a nap is just not an option, but you can increase your energy level in other ways. The first step is to realize that when your energy level feels low, it is usually not your *physical* energy that is low but your *mental* energy. There is a difference between being physically tired and mentally tired. Mental tiredness can happen at any time and in any situation. For example, you can be writing a report and suddenly you don't feel like writing anymore.

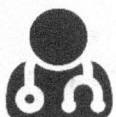

Skill Prescription:

1:1 Breathing

This easy technique can help you control your energy.

How-To: Try breathing in and out with equal counts. If you breathe in for 4 counts, breathe out for 4 counts. This 1 to 1 breathing ratio is associated with increased energy and focus.

Dose: Try this for three to five minutes. See if you can increase the number of seconds after a few cycles.

There are several other things that you can do to feel refreshed when working on a difficult task. Taking breaks can actually improve your productivity. It may be helpful to walk away from the task to another room for a few minutes. If you have time, you might also try taking a walk around the block or doing some stretching exercises. Exercise not only helps renew energy but can also reduce stress and make you feel calmer and think more clearly.

Call for Reinforcements

I like to think of sleeping pills as a last resort. If you have tried all the methods described in this chapter and you still cannot sleep, please ask your doctor for help. However, there are a few more natural products available that might do the trick.

Chamomile Tea

Perhaps you have seen Sleepy Time Tea at your local supermarket. One of the main ingredients in that tea is chamomile. This is a tea that has a gently relaxing effect on the mind and body and can be used right before bed.

Lavender

Lavender is an herb that is thought to have many healing qualities. The scent of lavender from a bag under your pillow, a spray, a lotion or essential oil on your temples or your pillow may help to calm the mind.

Music/White Noise

There are some musicians who compose music specially designed to promote relaxation. One of these I recommend to patients is Liquid Mind, but there are many different options available. There are also machines, alarm clocks, and smart phone apps that will make background noise such as waterfalls, fans, or waves crashing. Some people find this helpful in relaxing enough to fall asleep. If only I had recorded my first college history professor—talk about promoting sleep!

Melatonin

Melatonin is naturally occurring in our bodies but begins to decrease as we get older. Taking small doses of melatonin can help a person fall asleep, but will not keep a person asleep who wakes up frequently during the night. It is also best used occasionally rather than as a daily supplement. I recommend that you consult your doctor before taking melatonin.

More Serious Concerns

There are some sleep conditions that may require medical attention. Obstructive Sleep Apnea (OSA) is a serious condition that can cause drowsiness and other serious health concerns, including depression. If you snore heavily or if you feel like you wake up suddenly throughout the night gasping for air, you may have OSA. Other symptoms include feeling grumpy or impatient, being forgetful, and falling asleep in the middle of activities or conversations.

If you work nights or late evenings, you may also have special concerns regarding sleep. Our natural sleep and wake times center around light. When you sleep during the day and are awake at night it can be very confusing for the body. This can also lead to some mental and physical concerns, and people who work second or third shift often feel drowsy most of the time. Light therapy and keeping a consistent schedule may be helpful in reducing these problems.

Finally, many medications cause drowsiness. If you are feeling tired all the time, I would encourage you to review your medications to see if any of them can cause drowsiness. Talk to your doctor about alternatives if the drowsiness becomes a problem.

Looking for More Information

This chapter gives you some general information about sleep and how it can help you function better and experience less stress. You may have additional questions or concerns after reading this information. For more information on sleep, you can look at some of the books and web sites listed below. You can also check your local library. Sleep is very important. If you believe you may have a serious problem, please talk to your doctor as soon as possible. Don't lose another night of good rest. Sweet dreams!

Books

The Harvard Medical School Guide to a Good Night's Sleep, by Lawrence Epstein and Steven Mardon (McGraw-Hill, 2006).

No More Sleepless Nights Workbook, by Peter Hauri and Murray Jarman (John Wiley & Sons, 2000).

Healing Night: The Science and Spirit of Sleeping, Dreaming and Awakening, by Rubin Naiman (Syren, 2005).

The No-Cry Sleep Solution for Toddlers and Preschoolers: Gentle Ways to Stop Bedtime Battles and Improve Your Child's Sleep, by Elizabeth Pantley (McGraw-Hill, 2005).

Audiobooks

Healthy Sleep: Fall Asleep Easily, Sleep More Deeply, Sleep Through the Night, Wake Up Refreshed, by Andrew Weil and Rubin Naiman (Sounds True, 2007).

Internet

www.sleepfoundation.org

✓ WELL TO DO LIST
Rest Is Best

How much sleep do you usually get each night?

_____

Do you feel that is enough sleep?

_____

If not, what negative consequences are you experiencing due to lack of sleep?

_____

Which issues do you struggle with? *(Circle all that apply)*

    Falling asleep

    Staying asleep

    Frequent waking

    Waking up too early

What do you think causes these issues?

_____

Do you believe you may have sleep apnea?

_____

Do you work evening or night shifts?

_____

Are you taking any medications that may be causing daytime drowsiness or difficulty sleeping?
(Discuss this with your doctor)

_____

Choose two or three things you can try in the next two weeks to improve your sleep:

☐ Limit awake time in bed /
Get out of bed when not tired

☐ Reduce alcohol consumption

☐ Get on a regular sleep schedule

☐ Stop smoking

☐ Establish a regular exercise routine

☐ Take a warm bath before bed

☐ Keep the bedroom quiet

☐ Establish a bedtime routine

☐ Adjust the temperature
of the room

☐ Remove TV and other lighted
screens from the room

☐ Adjust snacking:

☐ Stop watching news for a week

☐ Reduce use of sleeping pills
to fall asleep

☐ Lavender

☐ Reduce use of caffeine

☐ Relaxing music/White noise

☐ Use relaxation exercises:
Progressive Muscle Relaxation Mattress
Yoga
Visualization
Deep Breathing
Mind Games

☐ Chamomile tea

☐ Melatonin
(Discuss this with your doctor)

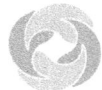

CHAPTER 8

Pain Management

A FEW MONTHS AGO WHILE DOING YOGA, I STARTED TO NOTICE that my shoulder felt a little tight. I was in a hurry and wanted to get through my practice, so I ignored my body's early warning signs. Suddenly, I fell to the floor as a sharp pain sliced up my shoulder. I couldn't move. I could barely breathe. My husband was terrified when he found me on the floor crying.

My shoulder has given me problems for years. I think it started when I was carrying enormous books on the train to graduate school. When life gets busy, it's my shoulder that reminds me that I'm doing too much. My shoulder reminds me if I have not been doing my yoga regularly. It also reminds me when I need to back off a little and let my body rest.

Years ago, my back served as that reminder. I started to feel some persistent pain in my lower back that radiated down to my right hip. I ignored it for seven months. As it progressed, I became unable to tie my shoes without terrible pain. I was only 24 years old. I went to a surgeon who told me to rest and gave me several prescriptions. I decided to get back to doing yoga instead. I joined a nearby yoga studio and within a month the pain was gone.

There's not one simple answer for how to deal with this kind of pain. For me, yoga keeps my back pain-free, but some positions can irritate my shoulder. Weight lifting has built up the muscles around my shoulder, but can irritate my back if I don't pay attention to form. What's a gal to do?

Dealing with Chronic Pain

Sometimes we have pain related to an injury or short-term illness. After a short time, or a simple procedure, or a few ibuprofen, the pain goes away. That's the easier kind of pain. The harder kind is chronic pain that never goes away. It might get better and worse at different times, but it does not seem to heal fully. Chronic pain is one of the most widely reported health problems in our society today.

The best way to manage pain is to deal with it before it becomes a big problem. Notice and take action when you are feeling that little tightness in the back, or a mild tension or discomfort. You can make your body stronger, more coordinated, and healthier with good habits that will keep you feeling comfortable and pain-free.

Even if you are good about trying to catch things early, almost everyone will have some kind of chronic pain, lasting longer than 3 months, at some time. While the solutions will vary by individual, the following practices have helped many people reduce or even cure chronic pain without expensive surgery or medication.

Walking and Movement

I know what you're thinking. You're wondering how you are going to walk when you are in pain. It's a fair question. I have many patients who tell me that they cannot walk because of arthritis. In fact, walking is one of the best treatments for arthritis. That doesn't stop my patients from scowling at me when I mention this, but it's still true.

For most people, simple regular walking can reduce pain and help control weight. Chronic pain can create a vicious cycle—because of the pain, we exercise less and move less. Because we move less, the pain gets worse. With walking and movement, it's possible to break the cycle and begin to feel better. Even if the pain is in your feet or legs, or you cannot walk, movement remains the most important thing you can do for your health. I talk more about this in Chapter 5.

Lots of people tell me that they cannot exercise because they are in pain. Sometimes this is true. However, experts say that the best way to deal with chronic pain is to get moving. This does not mean you have to join an aerobics class and buy a lot of spandex clothing, but it does mean that your body needs to be in motion. This can start with simple activities like walking. If that is too painful, then start moving the parts of your body that do feel good. If your back hurts then maybe you can start using an arm bike. If your shoulder hurts, maybe riding a stationary bike would be a good start. Try to build up to moving the parts of your body that are in pain.

A good physical therapist can help you with your first attempts at exercise. Ask your doctor for a recommendation. Physical therapists can help you identify exercises that increase flexibility and do them in ways that are safe for you. They also have great tools to help manage pain in between sessions and during your treatments. In many cases, these treatments can help reduce the amount of pain medication you will need and may help you avoid surgery. That sounds pretty good to me.

Weight Lifting

Weight lifting is another exercise that can help to manage pain. I used to worry that lifting weights would make me look like a bulky body builder. It turns out you would have to put in a *lot* of weight time before that would happen. In fact, that kind of bulk takes a tremendous amount of work and discipline. Starting with small weights can help to strengthen muscles around the trouble spot. It can also make you stronger in general, which can help to prevent injuries. An added benefit is increased muscle, and muscle burns fat even when you are resting. It is possible to make injuries worse with weight lifting, so consult your doctor first. This is another area where physical therapists and personal trainers can help.

Yoga

Yoga is magic! Well, it sure seems to work like magic, improving many kinds of physical ailments, including pain. Some of the stories of people healing themselves and restoring a pain-free life with yoga seem miraculous, but they are true.

Keeping the body loose and flexible is a great way to avoid injuries. A physical therapist, personal trainer, fitness instructor, or video can teach you how to do some simple, yoga-based stretches. My recommendation is to seek out a class in your area. Many community centers offer courses for an affordable price.

Yoga is best learned from an experienced and thoughtful teacher. There are funny names for different poses and a teacher can help you make sense of them and try them safely. In addition, many of us are really not aware of what is going on in our bodies when we attempt a pose. You might swear that your back arm is straight as a board when it is actually angled towards the floor. A yoga instructor can catch these things and help you to understand your body better.

The guidance and adjustments from a teacher can help you notice posture issues that may be causing pain. For example, many people put their head forward and point their chin ahead of them. This can cause headaches as blood flow is interrupted to the brain. Other people stand with one foot or hip always in front. Over time this can cause hip, back and shoulder pain. Other people turn their feet in funny ways, which can cause foot, ankle, and knee pain. Adjusting your posture to correct these areas can make a huge difference. Yoga can also cultivate an awareness of pain or tension in its early stages so you can care for the area before it becomes a problem.

Yoga can be intimidating to a lot of people. People always tell me they can't do yoga because they are too stiff or inflexible. Well, honey, that's why you need yoga! I have been in hundreds of yoga classes with people who were surely made of rubber. They bend and flex in every direction and honestly I am not sure they get as much benefit as someone who struggles to touch their toes. In my experience, it is the struggle and the slow progress that is the magic of yoga. The first day, your toes feel like they are a mile away. You can't even imagine reaching them. Slowly, your body opens and over time you sink deeper into the pose and one day you meet your toes for the first time and you feel like you conquered the world. In the process, you are letting go of muscle tightness and preventing future injury.

Yoga also helps people control their diet. This surprised me. As I started to do yoga more often, I also started to notice the effect different foods had on my body. For example, I found that I was less flexible and felt heavier on the days after eating a lot of meat. I also noticed that I felt more tired the day after having a few drinks with friends. I don't plan on giving up wine and burgers entirely, but I do make different choices now and consume these things in moderation.

Yoga has also taught me self-discipline and self-control. When I am holding a pose, I might think to myself, "I could not possibly hold this pose a second longer," but then the instructor provides a little encouragement and I manage to continue on. I think this is like the challenges all of us face in daily life. We think we cannot bear another minute of a difficult situation, and we might use things like anger, alcohol, drugs, or food to cope. Yoga teaches you that you are much stronger than you think you are and you don't need these things to cope anymore.

Watching Your Weight

A great way to reduce pain, especially in joints, is to lose weight. If you know that you are overweight, then taking steps to lose weight will likely make a huge difference in reducing pain. Take some time to review the chapters on eating (Chapters 3 and 4) and exercise (Chapter 5) in this book to find ideas for how to get started.

I have worked with so many people who started off very overweight. They had aches and pains everywhere and truly believed they were doomed to live the rest of their lives as prisoners of their bodies. I have also seen some small changes make a big difference. You don't have to stay locked inside a body that is literally and figuratively weighing you down.

Supplements

There are several vitamins and supplements I would recommend if you are experiencing chronic pain or if you have a family history of chronic pain. Let's start with calcium, which most people have heard of. Calcium is essential for bone strength and, since our body doesn't make it, we have to get it from foods or supplements. You can get calcium from milk, leafy green vegetables and some nuts, such as almonds. Without calcium, our bones get porous and weak. This condition is known as osteoporosis. With proper amounts of calcium, bones are strong and sturdy and are less likely to break when you trip, fall, or bump into something.

Calcium needs a little help to get into the bones. Vitamin D and magnesium can help calcium absorb into the body. There are also some things that can get in calcium's way. Some experts believe that the phosphorus and caffeine in soda can reduce the amount of calcium getting to your bones. You may want to consider cutting down on soda and caffeinated drinks if osteoporosis runs in your family or you are concerned about bone strength.

Many experts in nutrition point to *inflammation* as another cause of chronic pain. The average American's diet is full of foods that cause inflammation and irritation, and can cause arthritis and other aches and pains. See Chapter 4 for more details on this. Omega-3 fatty acids found in fish oil, flax seeds, and other sources, can help to reduce inflammation over time.

Glucosamine and chondroitin are chemicals that are part of normal <u>cartilage</u>, which serves as a cushion between the bones in a joint. Although many people take these supplements alone or together to help with conditions such as osteoarthritis, the results are mixed. You should talk to your doctor about taking these or any other supplements. Be aware that glucosamine is made from shellfish and should not be taken if you have shellfish allergies.

Food Allergies

Gluten

There are some foods that can cause pain and make certain chronic pain conditions worse. Gluten is an often-overlooked culprit in some arthritis symptoms. Gluten is a protein composite found in wheat, rye, and barley, and it gives dough its elasticity and chewy texture. Gluten is also found in many foods and even beauty products. Although a true gluten allergy or celiac disease is rare, many people have gluten intolerance which can cause various symptoms, including arthritis, pain, digestion issues, fatigue, asthma, skin rashes, migraines, and diarrhea.

After a year without gluten, my own mother-in-law found that she was able to get on the floor easily and play with her grandkids. She had more energy and did not need her previously required ibuprofen after doing yard work. This has been a huge change, helping her to feel younger, more active, and more able to live her life exactly as she pleases.

Some health professionals are now recommending a trial of a gluten-free diet for chronic pain. It can be tricky because gluten hides out in numerous foods that you would not suspect. If you would like to try going gluten-free, I suggest you work with your doctor or a nutritionist who is knowledgeable about this topic. I recommend reading *Living Gluten-Free for Dummies,* by Danna Korn, and *The G-Free Diet: A Gluten-Free Survival Guide,* by Elizabeth Hasselbeck, for more information. I am especially fond of the recipes, photos, and advice from the Gluten-Free Goddess web site (<u>glutenfreegoddess.blogspot.com/</u>). This blog is full of delicious recipes that will make your tummy extremely happy. She also divides recipes by other dietary needs and preferences such as vegetarian, vegan, and dairy-free.

Nightshades

We have always been told to eat our vegetables, but some people may need to take a look at *which* vegetables they are eating. Nightshades are a family of vegetables including eggplant, potatoes, peppers, tomatoes, tomatillos, pimentos, paprika, and cayenne pepper—all my favorite vegetables. In some alternative schools of healing such as Ayurveda, practitioners believe this vegetable family can cause inflammation in the joints which may worsen pains you already have. Some people are more sensitive than others, and in those with high sensitivity, nightshades may cause stomach upset, digestion issues, joint pain and even muscle tremors. Some doctors recommend that patients with GERD, gout, and arthritis avoid nightshades.

Progressive Muscle Relaxation

When a person is in pain, he or she often walks around in a very tense posture. As other muscles tighten, this makes the original pain worse and may cause new areas of pain. *Progressive Muscle Relaxation* (PMR) is a common practice that is very helpful for learning the difference between tight and relaxed. It's a method of relaxing each body part one by one and letting go of tension. This practice is recommended by many healthcare practitioners as a way to increase awareness of when you are holding tension in the body. It's also a good daily practice to manage and even prevent chronic pain.

The basic idea is that you start at one end of the body and work your way to the other end by tensing and then releasing each body part. This allows the body to let go of tension, and it gives you time to focus your attention on truly relaxing the body. I prefer to start with the feet because I think it is easier, since most of us are not holding a lot of toe tension. With each inhale, you will hold a body part very tightly. Each time you release a muscle, you also release the breath and soften the body part. When you first start this practice you may feel silly, but you'll soon see a difference.

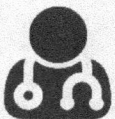 Skill Prescription:

Progressive Muscle Relaxation (PMR) Exercise

1. Sit or lie quietly with the legs and arms uncrossed.
2. As you inhale, tighten the toes by curling them under.
3. As you exhale, release all tension from the toes.
4. On the next inhale, tighten the feet.
5. As you exhale, release all tension from the feet.
6. Inhale and tighten the calves. Exhale and release.
7. Inhale and tighten the thighs. Exhale and release.

8. Inhale and tighten the buttocks. Exhale and release.

9. Inhale and tighten the stomach. Exhale and release.

10. Inhale and tighten the chest. Exhale and release.

11. Inhale and tighten the shoulders. Exhale and release.

12. Inhale and tighten the upper back. Exhale and release.

13. Inhale and tighten the middle back. Exhale and release.

14. Inhale and tighten the lower back. Exhale and release.

15. Inhale and tighten the neck. Exhale and release.

16. Inhale and tighten the jaw. Exhale and release.

17. Inhale and squeeze the eyes shut. Exhale and release.

18. Inhale and wrinkle the forehead. Exhale and release.

19. Take a moment to scan the body from head to toe and notice if there is any remaining tension. If there is, repeat the process in those areas.

20. Take a few more breaths to enjoy feeling relaxed and comfortable.

There are times when PMR is more difficult. If you have severe chronic pain or have lost sensation or movement in a particular body part, PMR may be uncomfortable, challenging and even painful. In this case, I recommend *Passive Muscle Relaxation*. In this practice you will just breathe into each body part. You can imagine it filling with air, then allowing it to soften as much as possible on the exhale, like allowing a balloon to deflate. This eliminates the need to tighten and tense the body. I also prefer this method when I am trying to fall asleep.

Hypnosis/Guided Imagery

Hypnosis and guided imagery can help you to learn to relax at a deeper level. The mind is a very powerful tool, and these practices can help you to use the mind to heal the body. Your brain is like a pharmacy full of hormones and chemicals that are effective at treating pain. There is an abundance of natural painkillers already within you. Using the imagination combined with deep relaxation can help you to harness these painkillers and heal yourself. The results can be amazing, and these painkillers have no negative side effects. You don't even have to wait in line at the pharmacy and there is no co-pay!

My favorite method of managing pain with guided imagery is to use color. Give your pain a color. It should be a color that you find unpleasant. Now choose a color that you find relaxing. After a period of relaxation using progressive or passive muscle relaxation, you can imagine that you are surrounded by the pleasant color. Each time you breathe in, this pleasant and healing color enters the body and goes to the site of pain. You can imagine that the pleasant color washes, blows, or wipes away the unpleasant color. As you exhale, the unpleasant pain color can blow, drift, wash, or crumble away. The point is to make the image personal. Many of my patients feel great relief after using this method, and the relief often lasts for some time.

You can find many recordings of relaxation for pain management online. Below are some resources to begin practicing:

- www.howtocopewithpain.org/resources/guided-imagery.html
- www.healingchronicpain.org/content/relax/default.asp

Creating Balance

In most cases there is not one method that will wipe away all your pain. The ideas in this chapter are meant to be practiced together. Take your time. Try some of the methods and see what works for you. Remember, managing pain is a lifelong practice that will require discipline and routine. Make these practices a part of your life and begin to take control of your pain. I wish you comfort, peace, and vitality.

Additional Resources

Books

From Fatigued to Fantastic, by Jacob Teitelbaum, MD (Avery Trade, 2007). This book is a classic text for those struggling with chronic fatigue and fibromyalgia.

When Things Fall Apart, by Pema Chödrön (Shambhala, 2002). Drawing from Buddhist philosophy, Pema Chödrön writes about what we can do when we feel our lives are falling apart and how we can find compassion for ourselves and others.

The Anatomy of Hope: How People Prevail in the Face of Illness, by Jerome Groopman (Random House, 2005). This book explores how some people remain hopeful in the face of difficult circumstances.

✓ WELL TO DO LIST
Manage Pain and Take Control

Location of any pain you experience:

_____

Description of pain:

_____

Your current pain score:

| 0 | 1 | 2 | 3 | 4 | 5 | 6 | 7 | 8 | 9 | 10 |

← *None*   *Worst pain ever* →

Your goal pain score: _____

Choose at least two skills you can practice this month to help manage pain:

☐ Manual Therapy
Physical Therapy
Massage
Osteopathic Manipulative Therapy

☐ Walking
What days/time will you walk?
How long will you walk?
Where will you walk?

☐ Other Movement
List a movement/exercise you will do this month.

☐ Weight Lifting
What exercises does your doctor recommend?
How many times a week?

☐ Yoga

Where can you practice yoga?

When will you practice yoga?

Does your doctor recommend any particular videos or resources?

☐ Weight Loss

What is your plan for weight loss?

What is your target weight loss for the next month?

☐ Gluten-Free Trial

Does your doctor have any resources to recommend?

☐ Progressive (or Passive) Muscle Relaxation

How of often will you practice?

What days/time will you practice?

☐ Hypnosis/Guided Imagery

How often will you practice?

What days/time will you practice?

☐ Supplements

What supplements does your doctor recommend? (list below)

Supplement / Dose / Frequency / Duration

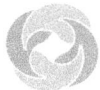

CHAPTER 9

Stress Management for You and the People Who Care for You

THE UNITED STATES IS ONE OF THE UNHEALTHIEST COUNTRIES IN THE WORLD, and most of the leading causes of death in our country are related to stress in some way. Heart disease, obesity, diabetes, asthma, allergies, skin conditions, chronic pain, depression and anxiety are all made worse or even caused by stress. Stress is the ultimate bad habit.

It's true that there is a level of stress that is actually healthy for us. There is stress that encourages us to perform better and try harder while still maintaining a healthy mental balance. Fearing my parents would ground me if I came home with failing grades certainly motivated me to study in high school. Knowing that you could lose your job if you don't show up may motivate you to stop pressing snooze on a cold and rainy morning and drag yourself out of bed and off to work.

However, there is a point where your body and mind can be so overwhelmed with stress that it never seems to end. Many of us experience this, occasionally or even regularly. We are still suffering the blows of one stressful thing while the next stressor is coming at us. The body has no time to recover. Over time, this can lead to problems.

We have a system in our body called the *sympathetic nervous system*. This system releases chemicals in our body that are needed in times of emergency. This is the kind of thing you might have needed in the wild when being chased. The heart starts to beat fast to pump blood to the legs for running. The body stops digesting food and takes all that energy to the legs and arms as well. Back in the wild you would have used that extra energy to flee the big, bad, scary animal, followed by some time to rest. It might be a few days or weeks before Big Bad came back. During this time, your *parasympathetic nervous system* would be busy repairing the damage and helping you feel relaxed and re-energized.

These days, it seems like Big Bad is around every corner. Whenever I tell people I'm a psychologist, they tell me about the relative or friend that they think I should see. But when I say that I specialize in stress management, they want to sign *themselves* up for an appointment. Sometimes we wear our stress like a medal, thinking that if we are not stressed then we are not trying hard enough. At the same time, the pressures and expectations of work, family, health and modern life are hard to avoid even when we try.

The Three Stages of Stress Management

Stress management is not really about managing stress. It's really about self-management. It's about managing our reactions and how we prepare ourselves to navigate through life. We need to start by recognizing that too much stress is bad. Then we need to make an effort to start making it more unwelcome in our lives. This takes time and work. I like to divide stress management into three stages.

First, we'll look at things you can do in the moment to manage stress as it closes in. Next, we'll look at things you can do after stressful events to repair the damage it causes. Finally, we'll examine practices you can do regularly to make you resistant to stress so that it doesn't harm you in the first place.

1	Coping	Surviving the moment, learning mindfulness and breathing, and shaking it off
2	Restoration	Repairing the damage after a big event
3	Prevention	Taking great care of yourself to keep stress from bothering you in the first place

The Three Stages of Stress Management

The First Stage: Surviving the Moment

It's an awful feeling to be trapped in a stressful moment. You feel your heart pounding in your chest. You want to get away but that's not usually an option. Maybe someone is angry with you or you're stuck in traffic and late for work. Perhaps you have a job that requires constant deadlines and late hours. Maybe things at home or in your romantic relationships are not going so well. How do you survive the moment? How do you keep yourself calm and healthy in the midst of unpleasant things?

Hidden Blessings

It is especially hard to want to be in a moment that is unpleasant. One way I have learned to bring myself into the moment is to ask myself, *"What is the hidden blessing in this moment?"* This habit has challenged me to really stop and think about what's happening and what advantages it might bring.

When I lived in Mexico to study Spanish, I had a teacher who required us to give oral presentations in front of a class of native Spanish speakers. This was extremely stressful for me, because I feared I would embarrass myself. Each time I had to speak in front of the class, I focused my mind on the benefit I would get—improving my Spanish—regardless of whether I made mistakes. By the end of the summer my Spanish had improved tremendously, and I was much more comfortable speaking Spanish with native speakers.

Recognizing the hidden blessing may help you switch your perspective, work harder, and maybe even enjoy an otherwise stressful event. At the minimum, it can help you to stay calmer and more focused on managing the situation in a mature and healthy way.

Fake It Until You Make It

I like to sing, and spent several years performing solos and singing with choirs. I always felt nervous just before performances. My stomach hurt, my heart pounded, my chest felt tight and I couldn't breathe well. Because of this, my first few notes were always shaky and pretty embarrassing. In college, I learned about relaxation techniques and I was able to trick my body and mind into staying calm so that my performances became more predictable and enjoyable.

It is really helpful to have a few tricks up your sleeve for those situations when you have to appear calm while you actually want to run away and cry. Maybe you work in customer service and people yell at you all the time for things that are not your fault. Maybe you work with people who are scared and are taking it out on you. Maybe you work with people who are mentally disturbed or just always angry. Maybe you are someone who hates public speaking but has to do it anyway. Perhaps you love to play music, act or sing but you get extremely nervous in front of other people. In these situations, you can trick yourself into staying calm and cool.

When you get nervous, your body starts to react with those feelings we talked about before, getting you ready to run away from Big Bad. All the thoughts that you tell yourself about the situation start to fuel the fire and make you feel even worse. That shallow, quick breathing tells your body that there is trouble ahead. The cool thing is that your breathing could also tell your body and mind that everything is fine, and you can use breathing to stop the stress cycle from causing damage.

Let's start with the basic mechanics of breathing. When I have people demonstrate a deep, relaxing breath, it usually makes me giggle. Most people look like their chest is super tight. They lift their shoulders with the inhale and sometimes even flare their nostrils, as if trying to get in that last bit of air. That does not look relaxing. Instead, deep relaxing breaths should fill the abdomen while you relax the shoulders. Try the technique below for a few breaths and see how you feel.

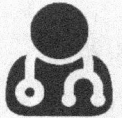 Skill Prescription:

Relaxation Breathing

1. Relax the shoulders, jaw and chest
2. Take in a breath so deep that the belly rises naturally
3. Try to exhale twice as long as you inhaled
4. Repeat for three to five cycles

Did you try it? Don't lie. Give it a try. The great thing is that you don't have to do it very long to get results, and no one has to know what you are up to. You can use breathing to avoid getting upset or angry. Angry people love to make other people angry so they are not alone, but when you don't cooperate they have to switch strategies and often calm down. You can use relaxation breathing before a big performance to reset your body to calm, cool and collected.

Time Out

When my daughter was a toddler there were a lot of *time outs* happening at my house. She was expressing all her 3-year-old glory with a temper that seemed somewhat familiar to me. We tried to respond by removing her from the situation and giving her a chance to think about her actions and calm herself down. I think I needed the time more than she did. On the rare occasions when she really got wound up and sent her cereal bowl flying or tried to hit one of us, I just wanted to scream. I started telling her that she needed to sit somewhere until "Mommy calms down." She eventually learned to remove herself from an upsetting situation until she is calm enough to manage it in a healthier way.

Why do we reserve time outs for kids? They are really brilliant. I encourage everyone to try it out. You may want to be subtle about it depending on your situation, as it might seem a little strange if a customer is yelling at you and you walk away to sit in the corner and breathe. You could say that you need to look something up or consult a co-worker. If you and your spouse are getting into a heated discussion (OK, an argument), you can say that you need some time to calm down so you don't say things you will later regret. These mini-retreats give you some time to clear your head and make decisions that you can be proud of.

Worries

I am an expert at worrying. I get myself all worked up thinking about what might happen or what I should have done differently. I worry about being late while stuck in traffic and I worry about how I will pay for various expenses.

What I have learned is that worry isn't terribly useful. It certainly doesn't fix anything. I've learned that it's best to stop worrying as soon as you become aware that you are doing it. Worry is like poison, and it will make you sick and unhappy. If you find yourself worrying, take a minute to ask yourself whether your worry is contributing to a solution. If it is not (which is probably the case), it's best to let it go. Use that energy to decide whether you can do anything to solve the problem, and if you can't, then accept the situation and move on to thinking about what *is* working and what is good right now.

Shake It Off

When I was in college, people started saying, "Shake it off," to others when bad things would happen. I started to wonder if you could literally do that. Can a person shake off stress like a dog shakes off water after a bath or swim? When I give workshops on stress, I ask everyone to stand up (as they are able) when I demonstrate this.

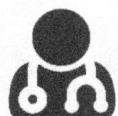

Skill Prescription:

Shake it Off

1. Stand up
2. Seriously, stand up! Go ahead. Don't be shy. OK, if you are in public you can save this part for later so you don't scare people.
3. If you're in a private place or around people with a good sense of humor, just start shaking all over. Really get into it. Enjoy!
4. How do you feel? Did you laugh at yourself? Did you feel silly? Good!

The point is to let loose a little. I think shaking after a difficult situation can actually help you relieve tension, breathe easier, and remember that most things really are not that serious. It's hilarious to watch groups of people do this together. Most people give it an honest try and almost everyone will start smiling and even laughing. However, you may want to wait until no one is looking. Or maybe you can explain what you're doing and invite others to shake along with you. You might be surprised who will join in.

Being in the Moment

Mindfulness may be our most powerful mind tool to deal with stress. There are times when life seems overwhelming because we are trying to handle everything at once rather than taking one task or challenge at a time.

Jack Kornfield's *Meditation for Beginners* includes an easy-to-read manual on meditation and a CD with lovely relaxation exercises. In his recordings, Kornfield reminds the listener to notice whenever he/she is "thinking, planning, or remembering." I think these are great cues to remind you what mindfulness is not. I'm really terrible at enjoying "the moment" or being present. I'm always thinking, planning or remembering what has gone wrong or all the things that I need to do. I have been on a date night with my husband and been wondering who I might get to babysit the next time we go out. I have been at amazing concerts thinking about who I have to tell about how great the show was. Being in the exact moment I'm in is very hard.

Maybe you find this difficult as well. Anytime you are daydreaming or forget what you were doing, you probably are not being present. The goal is to be *mindful*. This means that you are really focused on what is going on in this exact moment. I describe this by encouraging people to ask themselves not, "*Where* am I right now?" but, "*When* am I right now?" This gives you a reminder to notice what time period is occupying your mind: the past, the future or right now.

The Second Stage: Renew and Restore

There are times when, despite your best efforts, life is just difficult. There are moments you just have to survive, but luckily there are many things you can do *after* a stressful situation to help recharge your emotional batteries. These are practices that will help your parasympathetic system kick in and start repairing the damage of stressful events. All of the skills we just discussed can be used in this way, but here are a few more for your toolbox.

Progressive Muscle Relaxation

Progressive Muscle Relaxation (PMR) is a common practice that is very helpful for learning the difference between calm and relaxed. It is a method of relaxing each body part one by one and letting go of tension. It is also a great distraction from worry and stress. This practice is recommended by many healthcare practitioners as a way to increase awareness of when you are holding tension in the body. See Chapter 8 for detailed instructions.

This is a great practice to do at night when your mind is racing and you cannot fall asleep. It is also good for feeling rested after completing one project and before moving on to the next.

The Onion

Another method of relaxation is to imagine that your stress is like the layers of an onion. With each breath, you fill the body with air. Then, as you exhale, you imagine that you are peeling away a layer of stress like the outer layer of an onion. Then inhale again and peel another layer away so that you feel more relaxed with each breath. Keep going until you feel totally relaxed.

Power Napping

There are many people who take a daily nap. I am jealous of them and hope to be like them one day, because a daily nap is a great practice. It's natural to feel a dip in energy in the afternoon, and a brief rest can make the rest of the day much easier and more enjoyable. See Chapter 7 for more information on power napping strategies.

Rituals

Whether you are working full time, raising children at home, or retired, the day can sometimes seem very long. I find it helpful to have some relaxing rituals throughout the day to get a mental break. I'm not talking about lighting candles and chanting around tree trunks here. I am thinking more along the lines of a walk around the block or a coffee break. Each day that I work at the hospital, I leave my desk and join my friend Marty for a run downstairs to buy a cup of coffee. We catch up on each other's lives and laugh a little bit, and when I get back to my desk I feel more energy. The whole process takes only about 10 minutes, and it makes my work more productive. It's something I look forward to.

Some people use their afternoon snack as a ritual. Some people take a walk at lunchtime with their friends. Others stop at the same coffee shop every day and have become friends with the staff. Maybe you read every afternoon or sit on the porch to watch the sunset. Perhaps you weed the garden every morning or water the plants every night. You might consider a weekly massage or manicure. Your ritual can be anything you enjoy that makes life more fun.

The Third Stage: Prevention, or "The Best Defense Is a Good Offense"

Now you know how to recover when you are feeling overwhelmed and dominated by stress. That's certainly helpful, but did you know that there are things you can do to make yourself tougher and more resistant to stress in the first place? In the normal cycle of stress, a stressful event makes you feel more tired and less healthy. Because of this, you are less able to manage the next stressful event. However, if you can learn to manage stress before it begins, stressful things may not seem so stressful anymore. Below are a few ideas that will help you build your stress-fighting muscles and to make your life more pleasant in general.

Get Moving

Having a regular exercise routine is one of the best ways to stay calm and cool when life gets crazy. Exercise helps to burn off anxiety by using up the chemicals in your body that make you feel nervous. It can help you release tight muscles and it also distracts the mind from worries and troubles. Please see the chapter on exercise for more details on how to get started.

I especially recommend yoga and tai chi for exercise options that really help with stress management. These practices combine breathing, stretching, and strengthening. They can improve balance both mentally and physically and increase focus. These practices can help train the mind to stay calm and clear in difficult times.

Get to Bed

So many of us are not getting enough sleep. I know that I could probably use about one to two hours more sleep a day than I usually get. What about you? Sleep is vital to helping your body repair itself from all the stressful things you do during the day. It also helps you process the things you have learned and to feel focused again. If you are struggling with the length or quality of your sleep, check out the chapter on sleep for tips to get the rest you need.

What's the Goal?

I think most of us feel that we have a lot to do but we have trouble keeping it all straight. It makes things easier if you have clear goals and realistic timelines to accomplish these goals. If you find this difficult, then review the chapter on changing behaviors (Chapter 2) for some ideas on goal-setting.

Have a Little Fun

Getting things done is important. Accomplishing goals helps you feel relaxed and proud. However, it's just as important to schedule time for fun and to have a good sense of humor. Take time to laugh and do things just for fun. If life is always serious, you'll be much less able to manage when things get tough. Sometimes a laugh can help you put things in perspective and see that things are not as terrible as you first thought. Laughing also helps to relieve tension. If you don't have a good sense of humor, try to surround yourself with people who do. You might learn a thing or two and begin to see the world differently.

Assemble the Troops

Father Brian Christopher, a dear friend of me and my husband, spoke at our wedding. The theme of the speech was that we are not meant to be alone. He emphasized that in times of trouble, it is our connection to others that helps us thrive. This is so true. You need friends. You need people to talk with and to be rational when you have lost perspective. You need people to hug you when you are sad and to celebrate your accomplishments. You need people who support you no matter what happens and who will get you moving when you can't do it yourself. We are social animals deeply wired to be together. We are not meant to be alone.

Be good to your friends. Thank them for being around. Remember what is important to them and share their excitement and tears. If some friends move away either physically or emotionally, then find new ones. Keep your life full of people who make life fun and meaningful, and with whom you can be yourself. These relationships are a great defense against stress.

Forgive and Forget

My daughter received an adorable book from her great uncle David when she was born. In *Zen Shorts,* by John J. Muth, a giant panda named Stillwater tells stories that teach respect and patience. In one story, a young monk and an older monk are walking together. They come across a woman who is very angry because she is stuck in her carriage because the ground is covered in mud. She is yelling and carrying on as her servants stand helplessly, overloaded with her possessions. The older monk approaches the woman and hefts her onto his back and carries her across the mud. As he places her gently down, she storms on her way without saying thank you.

The two monks continue on their way. After a while, the elder monk notices that the young monk is very upset. When he asks his young friend why he is angry, the young monk responds, "You carried that angry woman across the mud and she did not even say thank you."

The elder monk smiles and says, "I laid that woman down miles ago. Why are you still carrying her?"

Every time I tell this story, people nod in recognition. How many times in life are you still carrying that grumpy woman miles later? How many times do you hold grudges and stay angry long after you should? It's time to let go of that resentment. I have heard people say that resentment is like drinking poison and hoping the other person will die. They won't, but you might. Resentment is poisonous and it can make you very sick and unhappy. Go ahead and lay that woman down.

Stretch Your Compassion Muscles

I really don't like parking garages. They make me feel trapped and angry. When I lived in Miami, the parking garage at my hospital had an attendant and it would take forever to get out at the end of the day. I became convinced that it was a conspiracy. I would be enraged when I'd find people digging in their cars looking for their ticket and blocking the whole lane. I would get so worked up that my coworker would tease me about it. One time she volunteered me for a live therapy demonstration suggesting that I needed to work on my parking garage issues.

The problem was that I was only focused on my own needs. I wanted to go home. I wanted to zoom out of the garage with no one to stop me and enjoy a stress-free ride home. What I had failed to do was think about what the experience of the parking garage might be like for other people.

Eventually, I found some peace by using compassion meditation. Compassion Meditation is an exercise in working the parts of the brain that help us to stay calm and rational, and help us attend to the needs of others. It is simple to do and has amazing results.

Although this type of meditation is very ancient, it has recently been studied using the latest technology by Dr. Richard Davidson of the University of Wisconsin. Davidson has shown that people who use Compassion Meditation show greatly increased activity in the part of the brain that controls impulses. In my case, it might help to control the impulse to scream or rear-end someone. For you, it might help to decrease fighting with your spouse or children. In fact, I have prescribed this to several patients who frequently argue with their spouses. Every one of them has reported that it helped them see the other's perspective and to stay calm in situations that used to infuriate them. Scientifically speaking, it helps strengthen your ability to think rationally about what is happening and form logical and appropriate responses that may preserve relationships.

Use the following Skill Prescription for Compassion Meditation to try this powerful stress reducer. It starts off easy to get you warmed up and then it gets more challenging.

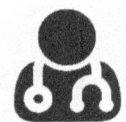

Skill Prescription:

Compassion Meditation

1. Take a few slow, deep, and relaxing breaths.
2. Call to mind a family member whom you love very much. Hold the image of that person in your mind.
3. Knowing that we all suffer at times, take an inhale and imagine that you could inhale that person's suffering. It looks like a dark, gray cloud.
4. Using the power of your own compassion and love, transform that gray cloud into a brilliant, glowing, white light of love and compassion.
5. Breathe out and for the next three exhales, imagine that you are sending that white light to your family member. With each breath, think quietly: "May you be free from pain and suffering. May you be filled with joy and peace."
6. Follow these same steps for
    a. A friend
    b. A stranger
    c. Yourself
    d. Someone you find more difficult
    e. A group of people
7. End by repeating, "May all living things be free from pain and suffering. May all living things be filled with joy and peace."

Honestly, this meditation has helped me tremendously. It has given me the space and calm to see other people's perspective and to engage with others from a place of love and caring rather than impatience and anger. I try to do this meditation a few times a week and should probably be doing it every day. I find myself saying the phrases above when I am stuck in traffic or if someone is being rude or inconsiderate. It reminds me that this person is likely suffering in a way that I cannot see and that he or she just needs love and compassion to start the healing process.

Did you know that most people see their own mistakes as errors made with the best of intentions? We are not so forgiving of others. Most people see others' mistakes as acts done on purpose and with bad intentions. Compassion Meditation can help us see that most of us are trying our best with the tools and experience we have. It helps us become closer to others and feel less lonely and sad. When we feel connected to others, life is less stressful and we are stronger emotionally.

Call for Reinforcements

There are a few other tools that you can consider when building up your resistance to stress. Each of these contributes to overall health and helps you to feel more relaxed, and can even improve your mood when you are overwhelmed.

Herbal Teas

Chamomile is a tea that has a gently relaxing effect on the mind and the body and can be used right before bed. Peppermint tea is thought to increase alertness and energy. It is also thought to help soothe an upset stomach. Choose organic teas whenever possible.

Lavender

Lavender is an herb that is thought to have many healing qualities. The scent of lavender from a bag under your pillow, a spray, a lotion or essential oil on you temples or pillow may help to calm the mind. It is also known to help with headaches. Try to choose organic products if using on the skin.

Fish Oil

Fish oil has omega-3s which decrease inflammation in the entire body, including the brain. Countries with low rates of depression often also have large rates of fish consumption. Taking fish oil has been linked with decreased violence in prisoners —imagine what it can do for a law-abiding citizen such as yourself! It has also been linked with better school performance, so I give it to my children daily in hopes that they can earn academic scholarships to college and I can vacation with the money I have saved. Omega-3s are highest in salmon, cod, herring and sardines. There are vegetarian forms of omega-3s available, but the body does not process them very well. Please consider taking fish oil capsules or eating more fish for the powerful and diverse effects it may have. See Chapter 3: Eating in a Modern World for more details on fish oil and why I am so excited about it.

Vitamin D

Here is another topic my loved ones are tired of hearing about. Low levels of Vitamin D have been linked with depressed mood and decreased energy. Vitamin D is essential for the absorption of calcium into the body, so people with low Vitamin D levels can have problems with chronic aches and pains. Unfortunately, many of us are low in Vitamin D because our bodies make it when we are exposed to sunlight and most of us spend the day indoors. Taking additional Vitamin D can improve overall health and may increase the effectiveness of antidepressant medication. Most people can safely take 1,000 to 2,000 IUs of Vitamin D daily. I prefer drops that can be easily placed on the tongue or in food. This is an easy way to sneak it into a child's meals. (Sneaking it into the food of cranky friends and family is not recommended.) Ask your doctor to test your Vitamin D levels and recommend a plan that is best for you.

Counseling

The plan above is great for dealing with the stress of daily life and keeping you healthy and happy. If you feel that you don't even have the energy to begin or that life seems hopeless and difficult all the time, you may need some help to get started. A therapist trained in Cognitive or Cognitive-Behavioral Therapy can teach you to stop negative thoughts and learn new ways of thinking that increase motivation and decrease stress.

Medications

Many people suffer from depression at some time in their lives, and depression can range greatly in severity. Along with counseling, if you are suffering from moderate to severe depression, a doctor may prescribe an antidepressant medication. These medications can be helpful in resetting your body and mind and giving you the energy to take control of your life and to begin using the great coping strategies from this chapter. It's important not to think of antidepressants as a permanent cure for stress.

Kick the Bad Stress Habit

Life offers plenty of challenges and causes of stress, but many daily events are not as important as we make them in our minds. Our own insecurities and bad habits can make life more stressful than it needs to be. Stress management can help us keep the daily stress level down, and deal with the big issues more calmly when they come. Start off with one of the ideas above and slowly build more of them into your daily routine. You will likely notice that life seems funnier, easier, and more enjoyable.

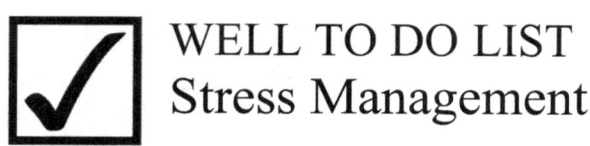

WELL TO DO LIST
Stress Management

In the Moment: choose one skill to practice for the next month.

☐ **Hidden Blessings**
Ask yourself, "What is the hidden blessing in this moment?"

☐ **Fake It Until You Make It**
Practice acting in a relaxed way.

☐ **Relaxation Breathing**
Practice the breathing described in this chapter.

☐ **Time Out**
Step away from stressful events in order to respond more effectively.

☐ **Reduce Worry**
Practice catching yourself worrying and stopping those thoughts.

☐ **Shake It Off**
Release tension physically and mentally.

☐ **Being in the Moment**
When are you right now?

Renew and Restore: pick one skill to practice for the next month.

☐ **Progressive Muscle Relaxation (PMR)**
Practice PMR three to five times a week.

☐ **The Onion**
Practice this visualization three to five times a week.

☐ **Power Napping**
Integrate a brief nap into your daily schedule.

☐ **Rituals**
Identify a ritual you can integrate into your daily schedule.

Prevention: pick one skill to integrate into your life for the next month.

☐ Get Moving
Move for 30 minutes total per day for three to five days a week. List your activity, where and when you will get moving.

☐ Get to Bed
Go to bed and get up at the same time daily. Write your schedule.

☐ Define Your Goals
Clearly define your goals in a measurable and realistic way. List them below.

☐ Have a Little Fun
Integrate one new fun activity as a regular part of your week. Describe the activity:

☐ Surround Yourself with Good People
Think of two positive people you can spend more time with. List their names.

☐ Letting Go of Resentment
Lay that woman down. List times where you will avoid holding on to negativity.

☐ Compassion Meditation
Practice this meditation three to five times a week. List when and where you will meditate.

Specifics for your selected prevention skill:

_____

_____

Reinforcements (discuss with your doctor whether any of the following may help):

☐ Chamomile Tea

☐ Medications
List Medication and dose.

☐ Lavender

☐ Vitamin D

☐ Peppermint Tea

☐ Counseling
Recommendations:

☐ Fish Oil

CHAPTER 10

Managing Illness

When life gives you lemons, turn them into chocolate and make everyone wonder how you did it.

—Unknown

Some of the information in this chapter is very similar to what you will find in Chapter 1: Managing Your Healthcare, but this is meant especially for those of you with a serious or chronic illnesses such as diabetes, chronic pain, cancer, MS, Parkinson's, Rheumatoid Arthritis, etc.

Three Patients

There is a patient I see a few times a year. Let's call her Anne. She's a tiny woman with a great smile and a cheerful voice. Anne has Multiple Sclerosis (MS) and she has been dealing with it for years. Anne comes into the hospital when her MS gets too difficult to manage on her own. She always arrives with a smile on her face. She has a great sense of humor and is a huge flirt. She makes everyone feel special and is a joy to work with. Anne has a supportive family, and the men in her family regularly carried her up a flight of stairs for years so she could stay in her home. She now lives in a senior apartment and is very active in many activities.

Anne gets down at times. She deals with a lot, and sometimes complains about her disease. She wishes she could wear regular clothes at home but knows she cannot undo her clothing fast enough to avoid the occasional accident, so she often wears dresses and robes. She would like to be a bigger part of her grandchildren's lives and she would like to travel more. She knows that her disease will get worse with time. She is not in denial.

However, Anne has made a choice to live life to the maximum that she is able. She has lots of friends, and goes to the theater and to her friends' parties. When she comes to the hospital, she calls everyone by name and remembers how many children they have. When she is in the hospital, she gets dressed every morning in nice clothes and wears jewelry. When she is home, she asks for help and expresses gratitude to everyone who helps her.

Sandra comes in often as well. She also has MS but is about 20 years younger than Anne. Sandra usually appears disheveled and depressed. She also has a good sense of humor but uses it to make jokes about how lonely and sad she is. Sandra denies having any friends. I have given Sandra information on MS support groups and social organizations as well as information on transportation. She has never attended these groups. Sandra is clever and talkative but she seems stuck. She feels that MS is a death sentence and often refers to herself as a freak.

Sam is another patient with MS that we see about once a year. Sam is a gentle giant. He is very respectful and polite. When he first came to see us, he was working two jobs. He is now on disability, but continues to volunteer at one of his old jobs whenever he is well enough. He is very devoted to his family and a loyal friend. Sam was recently able to stop smoking. He joined a gym and lost a lot of weight after his family doctor encouraged him. He takes the bus and walks to the gym almost every day. A few months ago he was named gym member of the month. He has also started speaking to MS groups about his own journey.

Sam is a proud man and still lives alone, although he is welcome to stay with his family. Before he was granted disability benefits, he went without food at times and had his car repossessed from the hospital parking lot because he was in the hospital and could not pay his bill on time. He still has trouble asking for help. When his MS gets the best of him, he sometimes tries to hide it from his family to avoid being hospitalized. However, he has gotten better at accepting help and he is always grateful.

If you have a chronic illness, you know that it's a constant struggle. When each day is just a little more challenging than it is for other people, you start to feel more tired and irritable, and life does not seem as fun. I'm not just going to tell you to cheer up, that everything is going to be OK, or that you should not be upset about your illness or illnesses. However, I hope this chapter might give you some ideas of how to manage those challenges better in order to feel more control and maybe more joy.

Some say that 95 to 99 percent of management of chronic illness has nothing to do with doctors. Well, then, who the heck is managing your illness?!? Oh, wait. It's you! That means you're in charge and are primarily responsible for successful symptom and disease management. But you have to choose to be in charge and to continue to make good choices every day.

Self-Management

Self-management is the ability of a person to manage all aspects of an illness from medications, symptoms and treatments, to the impact on family, work and social life. Many researchers believe that patients with chronic illnesses are healthier if they learn to effectively use *self-management skills.* That means if you learn to manage stress, what to do in emergencies, whom to call to answer questions, how to adjust your medications, and how to safely stay active, you will do much better than if you just learn the markers of your disease (like blood pressure, A1C, weight, cholesterol) and what medications you take.

We can divide these self-management skills into three categories: Management of Your Condition, Management of Your Relationships and Roles, and Management of Your Emotions.

Part 1: Managing Your Condition

Who Is in Charge Here?

If you have read any other chapters in this book, you might already know that I want you to sit in the driver's seat when it comes to your health. It's so important that you think of yourself as the head of Team Healthy You. Maybe you're not a sports fan and would like to take a business approach. I hereby name you the president and CEO of Healthy You, Inc. It doesn't pay well, but you get to boss people around!

Your doctor cares about your health. I hope your family cares about your health, too. Friends and co-workers are probably glad to help as well, but no one has the unique skills that you have to know exactly what you need to make the most of your life. If your healthcare provider or anyone else is working harder than you are, something is wrong.

As CEO of Healthy You, Inc., you must know and understand what all your "employees" are contributing. You will want to keep track of costs and benefits and be aware when someone on your team is not contributing. That person may need feedback to do his or her job better or it may be time for a layoff. You get to decide what direction the company is going and where you want to focus your energies. However, you are ultimately responsible for the company's results—and you get the profits. Your success will be measured by how happy, active, and informed you are. These results will depend mostly on how much you contributed.

This is not a company where the boss gets a private office and sits with his or her feet on the desk all day long barking orders. This is a company where the boss works harder than anyone else and understands just how valuable and important the work is.

Traffic Control

Our current healthcare system has become more and more specialized. Pretty soon you won't just go to the eye doctor, you will have a left eye doctor and a right eye doctor. We might even have a special doctor for each toe and maybe a separate toenail doctor. At the hospital, my patients often tell me that they have lost track of the doctors that come to see them every day. Each doctor gives you instructions and then a separate list of medications.

The problem is that many of these doctors don't talk to each other. If only there were someone who could help you sort through all this information to make sure that there are no harmful interactions with your medications, or to decide what's right when one doctor tells you to rest and the next doctor tells you to exercise.

Allow me to introduce you to your Primary Care Provider (PCP). This can be a family doctor, an internal medicine doctor, or a nurse practitioner. These doctors are trained as generalists and focus on all areas of medicine. Many of them even spend time in hospitals and treat very serious illnesses. Your PCP can help you review all of the information you are receiving and make sense of what's best for you. I like to think of a PCP as a guide who facilitates communication and explains things to you in plain English. Your PCP is like the general contractor on a construction project who knows a great deal about all areas of the project and can help coordinate all the specialized services that contribute to the end result.

Not every PCP is good at this. I encourage you to find one who is. When you have a chronic illness, you may put a lot of faith in your specialty doctors, but don't underestimate the value of the doctor who looks at you as a whole person and can help you put the puzzle pieces together in a realistic way. Sometimes the doctors may not agree. Do your research. Ask around. Get a second opinion. However, I would advise you to trust the doctor who seems to care about you as a person, tells you bad news when necessary, and who is able to talk intelligently about the latest research and provide you with more than one option to consider.

I know these doctors exist because I work with them every day. It can be exhausting to start over with a new physician, but keep searching until you find one that feels right for you. You are more likely to share important information and work harder for a doctor that you respect and like. If that doctor feels respected and valued, he or she will also have more energy and passion for you and your well being.

Know Your Disease

Step one in being a great CEO of Healthy You, Inc., is being an expert on the business of your disease.

It's so important to know what you are dealing with. What you don't know *can* hurt you and often will. Take charge of your illness by learning more about it. Go to the library at your local hospital and ask the librarian there for help. Consult the local and national organizations dedicated to your disease or condition. Talk to doctors, nurses, therapists, nutritionists, pharmacists and psychologists. Talk to other people with the same illness. Know what treatments are available, which treatments are proven, and which ones are considered dangerous or experimental. Also, know if your disease is progressive and will get worse. How will your condition change over time? How will you feel in each stage, and how variable are the symptoms from day to day? Knowing this is key to being ready to practice self-management.

Know Your Medications

Recently, a new patient told me that she had taken an anti-anxiety medication a few weeks ago, and that she had a violent reaction and woke up at night disoriented and agitated. She swore she would never take that medication again, but she could not tell me what the name of the medication was.

This is extremely important: No matter what medicines you take, you should know their names, doses and how often you take them. Keep a list of your medications with you at all times, on paper or in your smartphone, so you are prepared in emergencies. You should also know what the most common side effects are and if there are times when you should not take them, such as when drinking alcohol. Keep track of your allergies and times when you had a negative reaction to a medication. Keep a list of these medications with your current medication list.

Whenever a doctor adds a new medication, ask why and whether there might be other ways to deal with the same problem. Often you will learn that changing your behaviors would accomplish the same goals with no negative side effects or co-pays. If you have the financial means, you can also ask if there are any supplements or natural products that have fewer side effects. These products should be researched carefully as well—just because something is "natural" does not make it safe.

You should also consult with your pharmacist. Many of them have an advanced degree and have studied medications for years. These professionals often know more about medication than your PCP does. That is their area of expertise.

Pharmacists can be a great source of information. Talk to them; they like to help. It is lonely behind that counter. They can help you understand your medications better and identify problems that might occur when combining medications. At some pharmacies, they can color-code your bottles to help keep things simple or print out instructions in different languages. Some will even help you organize your medications into a pill box to reduce mistakes you might make. Often, they do this for free. That is so sweet of them!

If you visit a busy pharmacy, there is often a line of people waiting to pick up prescriptions. You may feel rushed because you don't want to cause a delay for others. The good news is you can make an appointment. That way, you can have plenty of time to talk to the pharmacist about your medications.

Know Your Treatments

You should apply the same level of research and questioning when doctors recommend treatments. I've met many people battling cancer who continue with chemotherapy and radiation without ever asking how much benefit it would bring. In some cases their chances of improvement are low, and the suffering caused by the treatments severe.

Ask your doctor about the risks and benefits of a treatment. If you are seriously ill, you should ask how much more time it might allow you, and how you will feel during the treatment. Before a treatment, you should know the side effects, what could go wrong, and how long it could take to recover. Ask when you can get back to work and other activities, and ask about alternative treatment options. Finally, ask if you will need a ride home. I once had to pick up a neighbor from the hospital at the last minute because no one had told him he wouldn't be allowed to drive home after his treatment!

Shaking Things Up

My husband makes fun of me all the time because I resist change. I love routines, and although I take up new hobbies and make new friends all the time, I really value having continuity in many aspects of daily life. I kept the same blocky cell phone for years after my friends were all using smartphones. It took me years to start using an electronic calendar instead of carrying around a folder-sized day planner. I'm not someone who changes things without good reason.

It's the same for most of us when it comes to health routines. We continue exercise routines long after we stop losing weight, we see doctors we don't understand or even like, and we take medications for years without questioning why. Many of my patients have been taking an antidepressant for 10 or more years but don't really feel that it's doing anything to improve their mood.

It is scary to make changes, but your body will go ahead and change without your permission. Pains might change places in the body. Fat starts to hang out where it never was before. Sometimes, the body even heals itself when we are not paying attention, but we keep taking the treatment or medication because that's what we have always done.

I don't want to encourage you to try every new thing that comes along, but it is good to be open to new ideas. It can be good for you and your doctors at every visit to ask, "So, what's new in the treatment of my disease or condition?" This will remind you and your doctors that you're always hoping to improve. If your doctor never seems to know the answer to this question, you may need to change doctors.

SOS

When you have a chronic illness, things sometimes go wrong. Sometimes these are minor problems, but other times you need help. Take the time to talk with your doctors about when to call the office. Know which problems can wait until the office opens tomorrow morning, and which mean you need to go straight to the emergency room. Make sure the people who live with you and care for you know this as well.

Keep an Open Mind

It's pretty rare to have a symptom or concern that only has one treatment option. For a headache you can take aspirin, Tylenol, or ibuprofen. You could also try smelling lavender, doing muscle relaxation exercises, face and head massage, sleep, acupuncture, or changes in diet. One or a combination of these might work for you, yet do nothing for someone else. That's part of what makes you special and unique. Whatever you choose is probably more likely to help if you are excited about it and believe it will work.

All these options are available to treat something as simple as a headache. Imagine what might be available for the treatment of your conditions. You might find that music therapy or art therapy helps you relax and gives you the chance to meet other people. You may discover that when petting a dog you have an increased range of motion. Massage might work for your sister but totally freak you out. Take the time to consider all the options available to you. Get creative. Ask around and keep an open mind. There is rarely one simple "cure" for any disease. Rather it is usually a work of trial and error, exploring possibilities and finding the right fit for you as an individual. This exploration can be an adventure and help you grow as a person.

A Few More Ideas

Many insurance companies can guide you to Self-Management Classes for particular diseases. These classes focus on all the things discussed in this chapter, in a setting with other people who have similar problems. Your doctor may host a group like this or the local and national associations for your disease may have suggestions. This is different from a simple support group, because it can help build the skills you need to manage your illness like an expert.

There are a few other things that can help. Eat a healthy diet. Giving the body fuel to heal is always a good idea. Take the time to exercise in a way that is safe and beneficial as well as fun. Talk to your doctor about this. Pace yourself—you don't need to do everything at once. You also shouldn't try to "catch up" the minute you start feeling better. If you do too much too quickly, you may overwork yourself and make things worse. Finally, take the time to rest and to get plenty of sleep. Your body needs this to heal.

Part 2 of this chapter discusses relationships and roles, which are also important in managing chronic illness. Take a break if you need one, do the worksheet below if you can or maybe just have a cup of tea. But keep reading when you can. Rome wasn't built in a day, and this information may take weeks to digest.

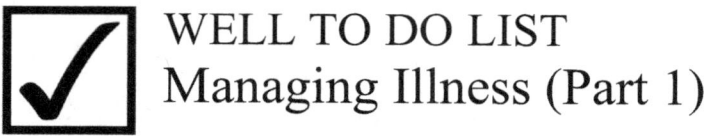 WELL TO DO LIST
Managing Illness (Part 1)

Part 1: Managing Your Condition

List your primary health issues (illnesses, conditions or concerns):

1. _____

2. _____

3. _____

When do you need to seek emergency care?

_____

List the medications, treatments and remedies you take for your health issue(s), along with their benefits and potential or known side effects:

Medication/Treatment/Remedy   Benefit(s)   Side effect(s)

_____   _____   _____

_____   _____   _____

_____   _____   _____

_____   _____   _____

_____   _____   _____

_____   _____   _____

_____   _____   _____

_____   _____   _____

_____   _____   _____

List specific resources that you will consult to learn more about your health issue(s): *Doctor, book, web site, friend, etc.*

_____

_____

_____

What are some additional medications, treatments or remedies you might like to try?

_____

_____

_____

Are there additional courses or resources available in your area?

_____

_____

Part 2: Managing Relationships

In my work at the hospital, I often talk with people about their shifting sense of identity when their health changes. Many people feel that they are worthless or a burden to others. If they cannot return to work, they start to wonder what kind of person they will be without the old routine. It's very likely that your co-workers, friends and family are wondering the same thing, but it's not for them to decide. You can take control of how you interact with and are seen by others. While illness can be a big deal, you are a person not a condition. You can shape your identity and, at the same time, help people to feel comfortable around you.

Rally the Troops

I had a patient recently who was an elderly woman. She had been in hospitals and nursing homes for months before she came to our unit. Her daughter flew in from out of town to be with her during her hospital stay and stayed by her side for almost every minute of her visit. As she approached the end of her stay, I began to talk with her about who would help her with various tasks throughout the day. With every question she replied, "My daughter will take care of that." It became clear to me that she was not comfortable asking anyone else for help. I wondered how long it would take for her daughter to be completely worn out.

When I know someone is in for a long period of health concerns, I always encourage them to reach out to as many people as possible and ask for help. What often happens is that people will rely on one or two family members and friends for almost everything. This will lead quickly to burnout for those people. It's a better idea to keep track of everyone who offers to help. In case you don't know what this sounds like, it's usually someone saying, "Let me know if you need anything," or, "Is there anything we can do?" Almost everyone who says these things *actually means it*. They want to help. That does not mean that they want to be your personal 24-hour caregiver, but they are willing to give over a little time to help you out.

Keep a list of those people. Take a minute to think about how those people might realistically be helpful. Some of them may be great cooks. Others may have endless patience for your children. One may be totally unreliable but always make you laugh, and maybe one of these people is good at doing hair and can help you stay presentable when you are hospitalized. Often someone from church can organize a prayer group, and a friend may be able to bring you good books or trashy gossip magazines when you are stuck in bed. Go ahead and make these assignments official. Keep it reasonable. People will be grateful for the opportunity to show how much they care about you in a way that honors their talents and skills.

When my grandmother approached the end of her life, she was hospitalized often and needed a lot of support. My aunt always did her hair and brought candy for the nurses who cared for her. My mother is a nurse, and she always managed the discussions with the doctors. My uncle took care of my grandmother's household maintenance. The grandchildren called and visited often, and I bought her simple comforts like lavender-scented things to help her relax. No one person did everything for her, and everyone was better off for it.

Be specific. Don't hesitate to ask. Be realistic about who can do what. Spread the responsibility across many people and no one will feel overly burdened.

Use Your Words

My husband is not usually very expressive about his feelings for me. His actions tell me that he loves me very much, but I have known him for more than 20 years and he has always been shy about saying, "I love you." At some point in our relationship I just started joking around with him and saying things like, "Did you cry today when you thought about how much you missed me?" or, "You love me so much, don't you?" He nods in agreement and then jokes that he had to hide his tears from his co-workers, and says he does indeed love me so much. The fact is, I need to hear the words. I like these things to be said out loud. Instead of waiting for my husband to change, which we all know does not work, I just cue him to provide what I need.

You can do the same thing. Not with my husband, of course, but with your close relationships. People can't read your mind, and they often can't begin to understand what you are going through. It's much less stressful if you can tell them what you need. You can even tell them how you would like to be treated. Telling people what you want or need, politely and matter-of-factly, is not rude. It's actually much more considerate than making people guess. It can help to explain the reason for your requests, so they know you are not simply being demanding.

If you use a wheelchair but don't like to be pushed, you can let people know. If you're invited to dinner but have dietary restrictions, inform your host and offer to bring something. If you avoid going out with friends because you are worried about bowel or bladder accidents, then let people know you would love to see them in your home and try to explain the problem as much as you can. Maybe you need a few days to be alone or you really want to be with friends but don't want to talk about your condition. Make this clear.

You can also exert control over how you want to be seen by others. I have worked with many individuals in wheelchairs or with missing limbs who feel that people won't look at them, and treat them like they are invisible. I think this is because we are taught that it's rude to stare. I encourage my patients to give people permission to look at them by looking them right in the eye and greeting them. "Good morning! How are you today?" That's a good start. "How 'bout them Packers?" (insert your local team here). "That's a beautiful hat! Was it a gift?" These comments let people know that you are friendly and open and that you are most certainly not invisible.

Strength in Numbers

No matter what disease or condition you have, I can almost guarantee that there is a society or organization devoted to this condition. Especially now, with the internet available for free in every library, you can easily find these groups. These organizations may offer support groups for you and your loved ones, education, links to research and treatment options, fundraising opportunities, and a sense that you are not alone in your struggles. It may even give you an opportunity to volunteer to mentor others or to become a leader in your community.

Community Resources

In most cities and towns, there are resources available at low or no cost to assist you with your needs. The YMCA has abundant services for people with special needs and they also have scholarship programs. For older adults, there may be a senior center nearby or resources for financial assistance. You may have secondary losses such as poor vision or hearing. Many organizations offer a variety of equipment to help you with these problems. Some groups rent or loan out medical equipment for a low fee or for free. These organizations are designed to help you maximize your potential and reduce your sense of isolation and helplessness. Talk to your doctor or do a search online at home or your local library to find resources near you.

Work

Many people are able to continue with work despite very challenging health conditions. It's helpful to inform your employer of your condition and help the necessary people understand what to expect. Ask for accommodations if you believe you can continue to do your job with reasonable changes. Make sure you understand the employee leave and sick policies in order to avoid breaking the rules. Also, don't be afraid to explore alternatives such as reducing your hours, working from home, shifting into other responsibilities or starting a new career. There are laws that can protect you and help you to keep your job. Talk to your human resources representative or contact the labor department in the state you live in. The Family Medical Leave Act and the Americans with Disabilities Act are specific laws you can refer to.

If you are not able to work, then get help with the application for disability. This is a terribly complicated process that can drive even the sanest person absolutely crazy. Make it clear to your doctors that this is your goal so they can help you obtain the appropriate documentation.

No Means No

It is so important to be able to say "no" sometimes. When you have a serious illness, you cannot do everything that people ask you to do. It is tempting to say "yes" to please people or to stay connected, but it is much more important that you care for yourself. If the first thought you have when someone asks for something is, "Ugh!" then that's probably your cue to politely decline.

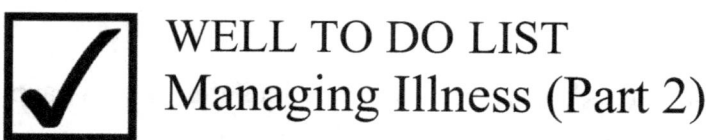

WELL TO DO LIST
Managing Illness (Part 2)

Part 2: Relationships

List some specific ways that people can help you:
Note: You can also go to www.carecalendar.org to organize a schedule online.

Ways to help	Who	Frequency	Day/Time
Example: Walk the Dog	*Jim S.*	*Daily*	*4pm*

List a few community resources and organizations that you can contact for help or support.

Organization Name	Contact Info	Services Provided
_____	_____	_____
_____	_____	_____
_____	_____	_____
_____	_____	_____
_____	_____	_____

List any changes at work that could make your day easier:

Accommodation	Who to Contact	Doctor's Note Needed?
_____	_____	Yes No

_____	_____	Yes	No
_____	_____	Yes	No
_____	_____	Yes	No

List three things you are currently doing that you can say "no" to:

1. _____

2. _____

3. _____

Part 3: Managing Your Emotions

Dealing with illness can be emotionally draining. I always tell my patients that I would be worried about them if they did not feel some distress about their condition. However, this doesn't mean that you have to be depressed and angry all the time. It's possible to live with health conditions and still be an emotionally stable person with meaningful relationships and the ability to help others.

Stress Management Education

They say the best defense is a good offense. Make sure that you know how to manage stress. Stress can make any condition or illness worse by damaging you physically and making you less able to make good decisions. In addition, having an illness makes life more stressful. Remember that stress management is a skill that requires practice. It is not something you learn one time and then move on. There are likely some stress management workshops or classes in your area. Otherwise, your local bookstore or library can help you find things you can work on at home. Take a look at the chapter in this book on stress management (Chapter 9) for more ideas.

Support Groups

Some people are reluctant to join support groups, but I think they have multiple benefits that are often overlooked. First, it is one thing for your doctors to tell you how to manage your illness, but it is much more powerful to hear this advice from people who know *exactly* what you are going through. These people may also tell you how to get through "real life" situations, including many that your healthcare providers won't know about or be able to describe because they have not experienced them.

Remember that support groups are not just for you. They may also be helpful for your spouse, children, family and friends. This will provide a place for them to learn how to help you and to cope with the ways their lives have changed.

Finally, my favorite part of support groups is that your peers can get away with pushing you harder and putting things in perspective in a way that is more direct and honest. If there are no support groups in your area, explore online options or consider talking to your specialists to see if they would be willing to host one at their offices.

Visualization

Take the time every day to visualize how you want to look and feel. Close your eyes and spend a few minutes imagining every detail of how you want to walk, talk, smile and act. How do you want to be seen by others? How do you want to treat others? If you have trouble at first, think of someone who inspires you and imagine what he or she would do in various situations. You can even rehearse the day's events before you begin the day and plan to be confident, happy, and motivated.

Do What You Love With the People You Love

As cliché as it sounds, life *is* too short to waste it doing things you don't like doing. Find time to do the things that you enjoy. Do fun things with fun people. Make the effort to plan social time and to set aside time for yourself. Take the best trips and do the coolest activities that you can afford. They say that money cannot buy happiness, and that's true if you try to buy *things*. But spending money on activities and experiences does enhance happiness. Choose activities that challenge your mind or bring you together with friends and family, and they are likely to make you feel better.

Volunteer

Here again we find that the research supports the emotional benefits of being active. People who volunteer tend to be happier and have a greater sense of well-being. Even if you are homebound you can make phone calls for your favorite political candidate (or even better, your favorite charity, because who likes politicians anyway). You can stuff envelopes and write letters to people. You can be a mentor to someone else who was just diagnosed with your condition. Previously I mentioned a patient who even volunteers at his former place of employment. This helps him stay connected with old friends and have a reason to get out of the house, while still being able to stay home on days when he gets sick. Helping others can give you back that sense of self-worth and can make a difference in the lives of others.

Laugh

Keep funny people around you. Be a funny person. Watch funny movies and TV shows. Spend time with kids. "Laughter is the best medicine" may sound too simple, but in many ways it is the truth.

Cry

My co-workers often come to me with concerns because a patient has been crying. They are often surprised when I am glad to hear it. Crying is a totally natural and reasonable response to dealing with illness. Crying because of pain, stress, fear, or exhaustion is not weakness, and it's not depression. It's coping.

If you need to cry, go ahead and let it out. A good cry can let out months and even years of frustration. Most people feel better after crying. However, if you find that you are crying often or you feel depressed, irritable or unmotivated most of the day for a few weeks or more, you may want to seek help from a good counselor or psychologist. Therapy can help you channel that frustration into skills that will help you move through it. Your doctor can help connect you with the right person.

Inspiration

If you want your body to run well, you have to fill it with wholesome foods (I talk more about this in Chapters 3 and 4). The same is true for your emotional health.

Surround yourself with inspiring things, people, places, songs and books. Read stories about other people who have been through what you are going through. Like a fight song at the beginning of a big game, you can listen to triumphant music that increases your motivation. Go to presentations or classes given by people you admire, or take a yoga class that focuses on healing. Find a religious or spiritual community that reminds you how valuable and loved you are. Fill your home, office and car with inspiring messages, photos, quotes and even scents that make you feel more hopeful. Make a space in your home that is peaceful and serves as a retreat to calm you when you feel overwhelmed.

Embrace Solitude

As my patients get ready to leave the hospital, I worry about how they will do when they are finally alone. The hospital is noisy and chaotic but it is also reassuring because you're surrounded by people who are there to take care of you. The transition to home can feel sudden and shocking. Take the time to be alone and to feel comfortable being alone. This is an important time for you to assess how things are going and where you might need to improve. Think of alone time as a space to renew your energy and to rest.

Practice Letting Go

When you have health conditions, there are so many things that you cannot control. There are times when you will have to accept that things cannot change or may even get worse. It's easy to waste energy thinking about all the things that you cannot change. In these cases, I encourage you to ask yourself what you *can* control. Can you do more exercise? Can you get out of the house more? Can you meditate or pray? Can you do relaxation exercises? Spend your energy on these things and let go of the rest.

Everything Is Negotiable

I used to think there were things that just absolutely had to be done. That was until I had a young child in daycare. The first year she was there, she was sick at least once a month. With no warning, I would receive a call from school that she had a fever and could not return to school the next day. All my meetings, assignments and errands would come to a screeching halt. This has also happened when a family member died and travel arrangements had to be made in just a few days. I have learned from these times that nearly everything can be rescheduled, and most of the time people will understand when you explain the reason.

Learn to set expectations ahead of time and let people know that your schedule can be unpredictable. Don't be afraid to cancel things when you need to. Your health is likely more important than whatever plans you had.

Practice Gratitude

I have a patient, John, who feels very overwhelmed by multiple serious health concerns that have lasted for decades. He also has a history of depression and he is a self-described pessimist. He finds it impossible to remain hopeful, and he often describes feeling pathetic and useless. John feels stuck in a very negative emotional space.

A few weeks ago, I started asking John to name three things he is grateful for. The effect was powerful. Almost immediately, John sat up straighter. He started to smile, and then the most amazing thing happened. For the first time since I met him, he started talking about how lucky he was compared to some other people like him. John had reached into the happy parts of his brain and he was feeling good. I have asked him to keep doing this every day and to try to think of three new things he is grateful for every day.

This technique from Positive Psychology is a great way to exercise the more positive and hopeful parts of your brain. These parts can get lazy from underuse when you are constantly dealing with health problems. Most people start by mentioning they are grateful for a friend or family member, and maybe their home or a pet. After a while, you have to get more creative, and you will mention things like the store clerk who always smiles at you or wool socks (for which I am very grateful here in Wisconsin). Pretty soon you may notice yourself being grateful for a wide range of different things.

This technique can be even more powerful if you keep a journal and write three new things every few days. This way, you have a great reference to review on the really tough days. As time goes by, you may even discover that you are looking for more and more things for which to be thankful, like a positive-thought scavenger hunt. That sounds like a good way to make the day more enjoyable.

Accept Yourself

I saved the best for last: You. That's right. You are the best! You are precious and valuable even with all your broken parts. You are talented and strong and the world needs you to just be yourself. We need you to take every opportunity to be the very best you there is. That is the best gift you can give to yourself and to all of us.

I think this quote from Marianne Williamson sums things up nicely. It's from *A Return to Love: Reflections on the Principles of a Course in Miracles:*

We are all meant to shine, as children do. We were born to make manifest the glory of God that is within us. It's not just in some of us; it's in everyone. And as we let our own light shine, we unconsciously give other people permission to do the same. As we are liberated from our own fear, our presence automatically liberates others.

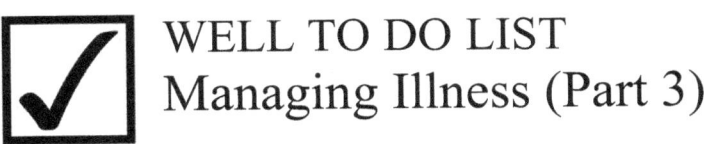

WELL TO DO LIST
Managing Illness (Part 3)

Part 3: Emotions

List some specific ways to manage stress:
You can read Chapter 9 for specific ideas about Stress Management.

Tool or Technique	Frequency	Day/Time
Example: Deep breathing	*Daily*	*Before bed*
_____	_____	_____
_____	_____	_____
_____	_____	_____
_____	_____	_____
_____	_____	_____

List one or more support groups that you or your family can join:

Organization Name	Contact / Location	Days/Times for Meetings
_____	_____	_____
_____	_____	_____
_____	_____	_____

Describe one way you can be of service to others:

_____

_____

List **things that you love doing** and that you can still enjoy:

Activity	With Whom	When
_____	_____	_____
_____	_____	_____
_____	_____	_____

_____   _____   _____

_____   _____   _____

Write out an inspirational quote that helps you stay focused and hopeful:

_____

_____

List three things for which you are grateful:

1. _____

2. _____

3. _____

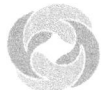

CHAPTER 11

Dying with Dignity

DURING MY FIRST WEEK AT A NEW JOB, I received a referral to meet with a woman (we'll call her Sara) who was described as "suicidal." Sara was 96 years old. She had pneumonia and became very weak while she was in the hospital. She mentioned to one of our team members that she felt it would be OK if she were dying. The staff member told the doctor and in no time I was asked to see this "suicidal" patient.

Sara told me that she had lived many good years and did not have any regrets. She felt loved by her family and had enjoyed her life immensely. She missed her husband who had passed away several years earlier, but she was not lost without him. Her family was very busy, but she saw them regularly and had many friends. Sara was not saying that she *wanted* to die and she was not suffering terribly. She was simply saying that if this was her time to go, then she was ready and willing. Suicidal? Not exactly.

In healthcare, we are trained to save lives but we are rarely trained in the skills needed to help people die with dignity and comfort. Let me be clear: I am not promoting physician-assisted suicide or any other kind of suicide. What I am saying is that sometimes it is a person's time to die. Sometimes the end is not a surprise and people have the ability to choose how and where they spend their last days. Many will choose to spend it with family instead of in a hospital receiving treatments that will not improve the quality of their lives.

Modern medicine is a miracle. We can save so many people who would have died years ago. We can improve the quality of many lives. We can treat the most serious diseases. However, we also keep many people alive longer to experience the negative consequences of strokes, heart attacks, traumatic brain injuries, and serious accidents. In many cases patients are able to enjoy additional quality years with their families and friends thanks to treatment. But there are also times when the best path is to allow a person to die with dignity and according to his or her needs and wishes.

This decision is especially difficult when someone faces a disease like cancer. I have seen doctors continue to offer expensive, painful treatments to reduce tumors when they know that the patient will die soon regardless. I don't say this to be alarming, but because it is true. Doctors want to save you almost as much as you want to be saved. They don't want to fail you. They don't want to quit. They are trained to keep looking for solutions. Families often feel the same way and avoid talking about death for fear that it will cause their loved one to give up hope. There can be great pressure on a patient to fight, to accept more treatments, even when the suffering is terrible and odds of meaningful benefit are tiny.

I pray you never have to face a grave illness, but if you do it is my hope that this chapter will help you and your doctor talk about your illness in an honest and direct way. I hope that it provides you with resources to make decisions about the end of your life well before it is close at hand. Hopefully, you can take the time now to organize your thoughts and wishes in a way that supports your needs and the needs of your family and leaves no room for doubt or confusion.

Plan Ahead

It's important to think about and discuss end-of-life choices before we face them. Often when the time for decision comes, the patient is weak or cannot speak. Planning ahead for end-of-life decisions is not fun, but a little bit of planning can make the process of dying much less stressful for patients and their families.

I suggest beginning some plans as soon as you are married, or beyond dependency on parents in daily life. It is definitely time to follow these steps if you receive a serious diagnosis, even if you are expected to survive for many more years.

Draft a Living Will

Also known as advanced directives, a living will is a document that you can put together to help your healthcare providers and your family know how you want to be treated when you have a serious condition or when you are dying. One of the best resources to help you organize your thoughts can be found on the Aging with Dignity web site at www.agingwithdignity.org/five-wishes.php.

The nonprofit organization Aging with Dignity coordinates the Five Wishes program to help people all over the country ensure that they have a legal document to support their wishes for treatment. The Five Wishes living will document asks five questions:

1. Who do you want to make your healthcare decisions when you cannot?
2. What kind of medical treatment do you want or not want?
3. How comfortable do you want to be?
4. How do you want to be treated by others?

5. What do you want your loved ones to know?

To date, this Five Wishes document is legal in 42 states but helpful in all states. It is also available in 26 languages. This document is very specific and can help you to think of things that you might otherwise miss. You can go to the web site and answer the questions and then print out a copy of your living will to provide to your family and healthcare providers. You can even email it. I have seen many situations when this was not done ahead of time, and it leads to confusion, frustration, anger and guilt for people involved. Taking the time to consider these questions before you are in a serious situation can keep your family from wondering what you would have wanted. If you cannot or do not wish to go online, at least take a moment to write down the answers to these questions and give them to your family and your doctor.

Weigh the Benefits

As I said before, doctors will almost always offer some sort of treatment. Treatment is a product like anything other. It is your job to find out what benefit this medication or treatment will bring you. That means asking how likely it is to succeed and how much more time the treatment will offer. Ask what you will feel like and what your quality of life will be like while receiving the treatment. You can also ask how much energy you will have, what medicines may help relieve side effects, and what alternatives exist. Make the doctor stay as long as you need and explain as much as you need.

In some cases, treatments may relieve pain or disability (palliative treatment) but will not prolong your life. This can be good because you will be comfortable. If a treatment prolongs your life but will make you feel very ill, you should consider whether that is what you want. Receiving treatment is always a choice, even when refusing may mean some shortening of life. You must decide what is best for you.

Make a Last Will and Testament

In her will, my grandmother felt the need to specify who would get everything from the china to some old supplies from my grandfather's dental office. She decided each child and grandchild's inheritance with great detail (and some spite—but that's a whole other book). The good news is, you don't have to be so specific. You can leave all your assets to one person or equally divided among a few people, and you can draft a legal will in as little as one hour.

Making a will can cost money. This may not be an option for everyone, but if you can afford to have one written for you, this can help to avoid problems after your death. If you can't afford to have an attorney prepare your will, there are reputable web sites that can guide you through building a will and provide it for less than $100. You can try legacywriter.com or legalzoom.com.

You do not want to leave it up to the state to decide who inherits your money and possessions. The state moves very slowly and a longer process will cost more. A good will can help you to make sure everything is legal and won't be delayed in courts.

Sadly, it is very common for families to argue, sometimes bitterly, over questions of inheritance. Sometimes family members appear near the end of life, just in time for a brief visit, before the funeral and proverbial reading of the will. For many of us, the thought of surviving family fighting over our estate is a nightmare. This is a very good reason to prepare a sound legal will, well in advance and with clear instructions, and tell the closest family members about it. This clarity is a final gift that you can leave to your family.

Funeral Arrangements

While a family is mourning, it's very stressful to make funeral arrangements. They have to ask themselves, "What would Dad want?" or, "Would Mom have liked this outfit?" If you are able, one of the best things you can do for your family is to plan your funeral. If you are ill, this can even help you to think about who and what is important to you and to view your life as worth celebrating. A funeral director can be very helpful in guiding you through these decisions.

One of my grandfathers was a funeral director. Naturally, my grandmother attended hundreds of funerals. Close to her death she sat my father and aunt down and gave clear instructions as to how her funeral should proceed. She also threatened to haunt us forever if certain songs were sung. We complied. You may not have such strong feelings about what happens at your funeral but taking care of the details ahead of time can allow your family and loved ones to focus on supporting each other through loss and sadness.

Hospice

My maternal grandmother suffered for a long time before her death. She had trouble breathing and became very anxious. She spent a lot of time in the hospital and receiving home care. As she approached death, the family decided to transfer her to a hospice center. After only one day she asked my mother if she had already died and was in heaven, because she was so comfortable and well cared-for. She ate and drank whatever she wanted. She had a huge window that opened onto a lovely view. She was surrounded by family and with healthcare professionals who honored her death as a moment as worthy of care as her life.

Many people think of hospice as a terribly sad place. In fact, hospice is a very nurturing and comfortable place where patients and families can be together and face death in the way that feels most appropriate. This can be different for everyone. For our family, it meant so much for people to see her comfortable and peaceful. In fact, my grandmother found a peace in hospice that was often lacking in the rest of her life. This effect was so profound that my aunt and mother now volunteered there in hopes of sharing that same experience with other families.

Thoughts of Dying

This chapter talks a lot about planning for death, but that does not mean I want patients to give up. On the contrary, life is valuable and we should make death wait until its time.

Many people who are suffering near the end of life have thoughts of dying. They may be terrified by these thoughts or wish death would come quickly so their suffering can end. Some even think about taking their own lives. It is one thing to refuse treatments or to accept comforting measures such as strong medications and sedatives close to death. It is another thing entirely to take your own life.

Despite what you might think, this action will not make things easier for your family. Your death will now be surrounded by shame, embarrassment, guilt and anger. Some loved ones might feel it is their fault. Others are left to tell family and friends what happened. In some cases, this may even result in an investigation and suspicion that family, loved ones, and caregivers assisted or encouraged the suicide.

If you find that your disease has affected your desire to live, or that you are thinking about or planning to take your own life, please talk to someone. Ask your doctor or nurse to recommend a good counselor. Talk openly to a trusted friend or family member. Their feedback and encouragement may be enough to keep you going. Practice the skills listed in the chapters in this book on stress management and managing chronic illness. Remember that your life is precious and you are precious despite all the challenges you face.

Additional Resources

Books

The Five People You Meet in Heaven, by Mitch Albom (Hyperion, 2003). This book considers all the little ways that your life is important to others. This is a good time to reflect on the gifts you have given to the world.

Tuesdays with Morrie: An Old Man, a Young Man, and Life's Greatest Lesson by Mitch Albom. Broadway, 2002. A true story of a man who meets with his mentor regularly while he is dying. Morrie is a man who is full of life even while dying.

Dying Well, by Ira Byock, MD (Riverhead Trade, 1998). A book written to help you manage everything from talking to family and doctors, to your fears of dying.

The Best Care Possible: A Physician's Quest to Transform Care Through the End of Life, by Ira Byock, MD (Avery, 2012). A great resource for healthcare providers. Dr. Byock writes passionately about the need for our culture to face our fear of death and dying.

On Death and Dying, by Elisabeth Kubler-Ross (Scribner, 1997). This is a classic work written by the co-founder of the hospice movement. This is a great resource for healthcare providers and loved ones. It focuses on the stages of grief and acceptance that most people experience when dealing with their own death or the loss of a loved one.

Being With Dying: Cultivating Compassion and Fearlessness in the Presence of Death, by Joan Halifax (Shambhala, 2009). A Buddhist approach to coping with death.

Being Mortal: Medicine and What Matters in the End, by Atul Gawande (Metropolitan Books, 2014). This is a newer book and is highly recommended by many of my physician colleagues. This book argues for a more humane approach to caring for those close to death.

Internet

The American Psychological Association has many resources including research, where to find a counselor, and what to say to children. www.apa.org/topics/death/index.aspx

The National Institutes of Health keeps an updated library of resources to help people in a variety of ways. It explains insurance coverage, medical procedures, and what to do after someone dies:

http://www.nlm.nih.gov/medlineplus/endoflifeissues.html

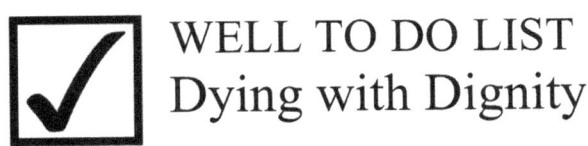 WELL TO DO LIST
Dying with Dignity

Living Will/Advance Directives

1. Who do you want to make your healthcare decisions when you cannot?

_____

2. What kind of medical treatment do you want or not want?

_____

3. How physically comfortable do you want to be?

_____

4. How do you want to be treated by others?

_____

5. What do you want your loved ones to know?

_____

Treatment Options

1. Do you understand your providers' treatment recommendations?

     YES   NO

2. Are there any specialists you are having trouble talking with about your treatment?

     YES   NO

Paperwork

1. Do you have a written will?

     Yes   No

2. Are there any special arrangements you would like your family to know about for your funeral?

     Yes   No

Resources

1. Do you need more information about hospice options in your area?

    Yes   No

2. Are there any other resources your provider can provide?

    Yes   No

Emotional Wellness

1. Do you ever think about harming yourself or ending your life?

    Yes   No

2. Who is available to support you through difficult emotional times?

_____

3. Who can you call in case of an emergency?

_____

Seven Secrets of Happy People

I ALWAYS FEEL TEMPTED TO LIE WHEN PEOPLE ASK WHAT I DO FOR A LIVING. If I tell people that I'm a psychologist, the response is often a look of horror. People ask, "Are you analyzing me right now?" They look at my husband with sympathy and wonder if my kids are really screwed up.

Why is this? I think it is because psychologists are known for figuring out what is *wrong* with you. They identify what's broken and try to make it go away. They try to make you less weird or strange to others.

But what about all that is *right* with you? What about what's working well or even great? What about identifying what's good and making it even better? Can we use your superpowers to compensate for or improve upon weaknesses? Of course we can.

I am greatly influenced by Positive Psychology, because I believe that it's a better use of energy to focus on creating positive feelings rather than just eliminating negative feelings. Positive Psychology practitioners might prescribe volunteering or a gratitude journal as a way to create happiness. We focus on a person's unique strengths and how to use those more effectively.

Bringing It Together

Throughout this book we have reviewed ways to create healthy habits in your life and to make small changes that add up to big results. We focused on the many ways that people struggle to get healthy and do their best. Now that you have looked at your special challenges and struggles, let's take a few minutes to review and to consider some habits that will ensure a lifetime of not only health but also happiness.

It's true that some people are born happier than others. They see things in a more optimistic way and things bother them less. Others are born with a more pessimistic or negative perspective.

These people are more skeptical and cautious. Both have their advantages, but there are certain habits that happy people seem to have in common. Let's review what you have learned in this book and take a look at how you can set some goals to increase joy and peace in your life.

Secret 1: Eat Healthy

Healthy food is a passion of mine. It is so important that I spent two chapters of this book (Eating in a Modern World and The Best Food for You) reviewing how food can affect your health. The bottom line is that eating real and simple foods that are naturally colorful and varied is a vital contribution to your mood. Processed foods have an excess of ingredients that cause inflammation, which leads to a variety of health concerns. One of them is depression. Healthy foods make the brain stronger and more resistant to stress and anger. In fact, eating a diet as described in this book is one of the best anger management tools available.

Secret 2: Sleep Well

In the chapter Rest Is Best, we review why sleep is important and how to improve your sleep. Sleep is a time for the brain to process everything it has experienced during the waking hours, a time to repair and renew before facing a new day. If sleep is too short or too interrupted, you will not have the resources to manage new data and input. If you are sleeping well, you are better able to process information, tackle novel challenges and solve problems. Thanks to your increased energy level, most people around you will seem less crazy and more reasonable.

Secret 3: Invest in Experiences

They say that money cannot buy happiness. That's not entirely true. When we invest in things like fancy cars, bigger houses, the latest fashions and expensive toys, we set ourselves up for future discontent. Someone will always have a better car, a bigger house, nicer clothes and more expensive toys. This competition puts distance between us and other people. It results in feeling isolated and envious.

When we invest our money in experiences, this is where the magic happens. Spend what money you do have on hobbies. Take a class and learn something new. Book a trip or play day with the people you love. These kinds of investments pay off big in feelings of increased self-worth and connectedness, and in keeping the mind young and active.

Secret 4: Get Moving

In the chapter Move It or Lose It, we reviewed the importance of movement in your overall health. A good 45 minutes of rigorous movement can burn off chemicals in the brain that cause anxiety, leaving you feeling calm and reasonable. Any movement that involves coordinating two sides of the body (walking, swimming, running, biking) forces the two halves of the brain to talk to each other. This conversation pulls energy away from the parts of the brain that are focusing on anger and resentment. This effect lasts long after the exercise is done.

Next time you are angry or frustrated, try taking a walk before you consider solutions to the problem. Movement will help you avoid "solutions" that you will regret later.

Secret 5: Practice Gratitude

Positive psychologists often prescribe gratitude journals to people struggling with depression. How often do you pause to reflect on what you are grateful for? This practice can improve your mood and create happiness and a sense of connectedness to others. Consider setting aside a few minutes each evening to write out three things for which you are grateful. Try to come up with three different things each day.

You will find that after a few weeks, you are more aware of feelings of gratitude. You may notice that you are thinking about what you might write in your list later that day. On the whole, you are spending more time in a place of contentment and peace than in one of resentment and anger. Not a bad pay-off for the simple task of making a quick list everyday.

If you want to really amp up your results, try telling people why you are grateful for them. Or make a commitment to say a special thank you to someone once a week or even once a day.

Secret 6: Assume Good Intent

How often do you find yourself thinking the worst of other people? Did you know that most people across the world tend to blame outside factors when they make mistakes? If you are late, it was the traffic or construction on the roads. We are not so generous with others. We tend to blame the person's intentions when he or she makes a mistake. When others are late, it must be due to poor planning or lack of responsibility. Suddenly that person's character is called into question.

This is a rough way to live because we find ourselves thinking the worst of people with very little information. This does not mean that there are no irresponsible or unpleasant people, but not nearly as many as we think.

The next time someone upsets you or does something that you find irritating, try to consider that the person may have good intentions. Give yourself some time to consider what those intentions might be. Maybe even get curious and start asking some questions to better understand the person's motivation. Perhaps the person who cut you off in traffic yesterday was racing to his child's first piano recital. Maybe your friend has not called or emailed you back because she is waiting to hear from her husband in order to provide you with a good answer. Could your co-worker be late because he stopped to get a sympathy card for another co-worker?

We don't know for sure. The point is not to excuse irresponsible behavior. The point is to weaken the certainty that makes you so angry and upset. This anger is not healthy and often not appropriate. Assuming good intent makes life more pleasant and it allows us to see each other as good people who sometimes make mistakes.

Secret 7: Serve Others

One of the best ways to feel happy and valuable is to share your time and talent with others. Finding ways to volunteer your time to serve others can improve mood, decrease isolation, improve self-worth, and create a sense of meaning beyond everyday challenges. This is also a way to use your talents that may not be expressed fully in other areas of your life. In addition, it can give you a chance to experiment with new skills such as leadership, organization, compassion, patience, and listening. Understanding the vast and varied needs in the world can broaden your perspective and increase your sense of gratitude.

You Are Perfect

These seven ideas may help you to feel happier and healthier. Each may help you become a more authentic you. In the end, what the world really needs is for you to be you to the best of your ability.

You are amazing, unique and beautiful. There is nothing more you need to be, do, or have to be happy. You are perfect just as you are. Yes, really. So smile, give love and enjoy every moment of this precious life.

—*Jynell St. James*

Best Wishes

I wish you, the CEO of Healthy You, Inc., great success in your endeavors.

Wait! There's More…

IF YOU ARE READY TO TAKE CHARGE, Online you can get the Well To Do List worksheets and Skill Prescriptions from this book as PDF files for easy printing, as well as a free mini-meditation recording and the links referenced in the chapters for easy navigation.

Visit: www.MySkillRx.com/WellToDoMore

I am super passionate about health and wellness, and I love to find and share links and resources – most of them free. To see the latest information please visit www.MySkillRx.com, and continue the conversation on Facebook, Twitter or Instagram (@MySkillRx). See you online!

Acknowledgements

IN THE TIME I GAVE BIRTH TO THIS BOOK I also gave birth to two children. After so many years, I'm pretty sure many thought I was just saying "I'm writing a book" to impress people but there were some people who stuck with me and encouraged me for all that time.

First, thanks to my parents Mike and Mary Dunn. They put a poster in my childhood room with the William Arthur Ward quote "If you can imagine it, you can achieve it." I grew up believing that I could accomplish anything if I was willing to work for it and my parents have continued to support my diverse (and sometimes questionable) goals and dreams.

Thank you to my husband, Ted, who pushed me to write this darned thing in the first place, read and edited many drafts, formatted the book, provided moral and technical support and countless other helpful gestures. To my children Naomi and Milo who are really spectacular human beings and have thus far consented to be featured as examples and story characters in my writing and presentations. I love my in-laws Nora and John for the free child care they provided, and my best friend Nina Laseau for always making me laugh and reminding me not to take myself so seriously.

Thank you to my first readers, Mary Dunn, Kathleen Jameson, Jackie Muirhead, Jill Roemer and Kristi Faulkner. Your feedback was essential to the development of my content and keeping me productive. Honor and respect to Dr. Dennis Baumgardner for giving me feedback in record time, Dr. Adam Miller (AriseMD.com) for focusing my goals and Dr. Rebecca Gallagher for her thoughtful comments and sticky notes. Thanks to Heather Ferber (BetterHealthByHeather.com) for some of the most productive lunch meetings ever. Deep love to Marlee Jansen, Rebekah Schaefer, and Laura Hulke (heartwoodhealingcollective.com) for finding more ways for me to improve.

I want to send a shout out to Jennifer Morales at Rex, LLC who is a great editor and made me make all the right changes that I was avoiding. Also, Jennifer rocked the foundation of my world beliefs by telling me that only old people put two spaces after a period.

A special acknowledgement to all the medical practitioners who read parts of my book, gave me ideas and kept me inspired. I wrote this book for you. This section would not be complete without a huge high five to the employees of Stone Creek Coffee and Collectivo Coffee Roasters both in Wauwatosa, WI. Without knowing it, you supplied the great customer service, decaf coffee and background noise that helped this focus-challenged lady get it done.

www.ingramcontent.com/pod-product-compliance
Lightning Source LLC
Chambersburg PA
CBHW081828280526
45789CB00007B/2384